The Original Metabolic Medicine's Cancer Cure

Dr. Kelley's

Do-it-Yourself Book

CANCER:

Curing the

INCURABLE

WITHOUT SURGERY, CHEMOTHERAPY OR RADIATION

by
DR. WILLIAM DONALD KELLEY, D.D.S., M.S.
with
FRED ROHÈ

author of
Metabolic Ecology
and
Dr. Kelley's Answer To Cancer

LIBRARY OF CONGRESS CATALOG CARD NUMBER **00-135-968**

CATEGORIES: 1. HEALTH & FITNESS 2. MEDICAL/NURSING/HOME CARE 3. NUTRITION
4. SELF-ACTUALIZATION / SELF-HELP

ISBN 09704290-0-2

PUBLISHED IN THE UNITED STATES BY
COLLEGE OF METABOLIC MEDICINE®

Distributed in the United States by:

New Century Promotions

3711 Alta Loma Drive

Bonita, CA 91902

800-768-8484 / 619-479-7852

Fax 619-479-3829

This book Is dedicated to Carol, Wanda
And to You, who have prayed for relief for yourself,
your loved ones, or friends.
You may tell them that
your prayers have been answered
And that all is well . . .
And so it is.

Advances in modern medicine boggle one's mind and are quite over-whelming. Yet illness has increased on every hand.

Since the medical communities, both orthodox and alternative, have failed so miserably in Health Care and succeeded so brilliantly in health-plundering, it would seem to justify one to investigate true health care concepts

CANCER
One must address the metabolic <u>process</u>.
Attacking the <u>product</u> of defective metabolism
leads one down a blind pathway to a dead end.

—William Donald Kelley, D.D.S., M.S.

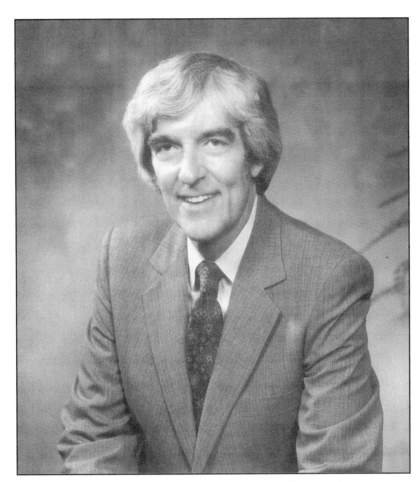

William D. Kelley, D.D.S., M.S.

Preface

What you are about to read may change your life forever.

When I was 11 years old, my brother Scott was diagnosed with terminal cancer at the age of 20. His story is unique because he was one of the 150,000 individuals lucky enough to find Dr. Kelley's book, ***One Answer To Cancer***, and one of the only 33,000 to actually go on the program. Today, he is healthy, cancer-free and living in California with his wife and three children. Scott's experience changed the lives of each member of our family.

For me, the effect appeared when I was older. Around the age of 19, I began to experiment with various diets. I cross-referenced my overall sense of energy and performances in running 10 kilometers to the diets I used, always allowing at least 90 days between any changes. What I found should come as no surprise to anyone: When I consumed a largely uncooked vegetarian diet, eliminated alcohol consumption and drank plenty of fresh-squeezed juices, my 10K running times and subsequent recovery periods were shorter than when I used a diet of more meat and cooked foods. In other words, my body worked better on simple fuels from nature.

The greatest majority of us are born in perfect health. Our health and aging process after birth is largely influenced by genetics, culture, geography and, of course, the foods and liquids we consume. These things are all that distinguish who will grow to be strong and who will grow weak. Why is it some people can live lives of smoking and poor diet and live to be 90 and others are susceptible to ill health and disease while living a relatively healthy lifestyle? The fact is, regardless of outward physical appearance, some people will become cancer victims and some apparently likely candidates will not. It is simply human nature that some bodies are innately stronger and more resistant than others. As adult individuals we have only one variable which is in our total control: Our diets.

The difference in lifestyle that you have led and your ancestry three generations removed are remarkable. We live in a world where air pollution is a daily occurrence; we work in jobs that are demanding in time, tolerance and ability to change and adapt; we struggle to balance our career, family, spiritual, emotional and social lives. Yet as a society we have largely failed to intelligently consider the fuels which run this remarkable human body, fuels that provide peak performance and keep our internal operating systems running properly.

When young, we feel invincible, immortal. Some of us develop habits and patterns in early adult life that prove detrimental later on. We eat too much dead food, drink too much alcohol, smoke cigarettes and take prescription drugs for any small perceived ill—all the while wrongly trusting that the regulatory bodies of society will look out for our health.

Well, in the words of a great songwriter: "I read the news today—oh boy."

Against the advice of leading doctors and scientists across the country, FDA commissioner Dr. Kessler approved the fat substitute "Olestra" for public consumption. Doctors across the country from Johns Hopkins to Harvard Medical School warned against the possible fallout from introducing this synthetic fat into the American diet for reasons which have been well published in the media (see Appendix II). Interestingly, most of the warning comes from the academic side of the medical science community. Why do you suppose that is? I'll tell you.

I have believed for a long time that the American Medical Complex and the Consumer Food and Beverage Industrial Complex have little interest in the prevention of disease. It makes far better business sense to let the population eat, drink and smoke to their heart's content and then offer seemingly high-tech and expensive methods for cleaning up the aftermath. In the United States, the food industry alone generates 500 billion dollars in sales: Bacon, eggs, milk, fast food franchises, soft drinks, fried food, dead food, overcooked food, sweets, treats and canned goods. We have gotten away from simple diets and become human garbage disposals. Sixty percent of the American public is overweight. Clearly the large food conglomerates are successfully marketing to an oblivious public. After feeding your body with dead and processed foods for 20, 30, 40 or more years, things begin to run less perfectly. We have overlooked the processing energy required to digest bacon and eggs each morning, that steak in the evening and the cocktails in between. The result is the current health crisis where one in two will have cancer in their lifetimes—not to mention heart disease.

Instead of educating the public on how our bodies function best, the medical establishment chooses instead to clean out those arteries with drugs and catheters, perform by-pass surgery or cut the problem out (or off) altogether. To be fair, the American medical community has done some wonderful things and made outstanding progress in the last 45 years. But it is simply not in their best interest to prevent disease. They are in the business of treating disease. The money is in surgery, MRI, radiation, chemo-therapy, research and examinations. The doctors do not want a disease-fee society any more than lawyers want a perfectly honest one.

This booklet is intended to provide an alternative view to conventional medicine in regard to 21st-Century disease—to profess prevention in healthy people and educate those who are ill. The human body is the most incredible of discoveries and perhaps receives so little consideration because we all get one upon entering into this life. We take it for granted until it cries out to us. Read this book and incorporate everything in it you can into your lifestyle. Listen to your heart and the voice within you and seek the advice of a trusted physician. On that note a word of caution: There are doctors who hold Dr. Kelley in high esteem and those who see him as a threat. Be prepared to encounter one or the other. The open-minded ones tend to be the former.

Finally, Dr. Kelley was aggressively persecuted and oppressed during his years of treating cancer patients. His success was unparalleled in conventional medicine. Personally, both my brother and my chiropractor went to him; both were resolved of their disease. Dr. Kelley has been forbidden to advise cancer victims. This book must carry with it a warning to all that it is not intended to be a cure, but rather a program to be used in conjunction with the guidance of your own physician for the resolution of degenerative disease. As the writer of this preface, I can say that the truth of Dr. Kelley's paradigm is both preventive and healing. I wish you Godspeed and hope that the truth will set you free.

Greg Stirling, Publisher
Vancouver, British Columbia
Canada

Foreword

Health is a wonderful possession, but it does not last forever — although most of us assume it will. It is not until we lose our health that we seek diligently to regain it. Often it is too late, and always too expensive.

It is the purpose of the College of Metabolic Medicine to help those who desire better health and who are willing to work for their better health. It is ever the objective of the college to point out the metabolic deficiencies in the metabolism of each person who has the malfunction, not to treat the disease who has the person. It is our desire to advise, teach, and counsel persons in such a way that they and they alone are responsible for their health. A doctor cannot "cure" you of anything. If you have a broken arm, the physician may set it — but only you — your own body — can "cure" or heal the break. Of course, during your lifetime you will need the help of many in the healing professions: The dentist, the osteopath, the chiropractor, the naturopath, the biochemist, the nutritionist, the therapist, and last, but not least, the spiritual counselor. Although these experts may give you aid, you must assume the responsibility of accepting and following their advice.

In researching some of the more complex disease processes, it became increasingly evident to us that cancer is a simple deficiency condition; we have proven this to our own satisfaction, and to the satisfaction of many counselees.

This publication is a simplified, condensed, practical application of our investigations and findings. We present these findings because there have been so many prayers unto God for a solution to this simple problem. To successfully resolve cancer, however simple, is a tedious and lengthy metabolic process, but not expensive compared to the "accepted" surgical, radiological, or chemotherapy methods and has proven very effective. It is our desire that this booklet be a helpful aid to many who are themselves or have lost loved ones afflicted with malignancy.

Introduction

A comprehensive defense program must recognize the existence of more than one potential enemy. Metabolic Medicine can handle other enemies besides cancer; it is, in fact, a lifestyle for peace or war — one that can keep you in an ideal state of readiness.

Over the last 30 years, the medical profession and the medical community have progressed to unprecedented heights and achievements in areas of reconstruction and surgical procedure. These professionals have worked hard and deserve every bit of the respect and honor they receive. They have done remarkably well in applying technological advances to their profession.

The medical community has centered its energies and advancement around infectious and traumatic cases and has all but conquered infections of all types. Surgical procedures and treatment of traumatic ills have advanced equally with control of the infectious diseases. In short, what the medical community does, it does well, unsurpassed in the history of mankind.

But the problems for which the medical community is so well trained and equipped to handle account for only a percentage of the illnesses in our society. In the balance of the cases involving degeneration or metabolic conditions, little hope is received. Through the years cancer patients have had such excellent results with Metabolic Medicine that they have brought other family members and friends for nutritional counseling. The range of diseases for which Dr. Kelley has planned nutritional programs covers the complete gamut of degenerative and metabolic ills, even some infectious diseases and structural conditions.

Dr. Kelley distinguishes between degenerative disease and metabolic disease in this example: Adult-onset diabetes is degenerative; childhood-onset diabetes is metabolic. Metabolic diseases can result from improper nutrition to the fetus due to the faulty diet of the mother during pregnancy. (It is widely recognized among medical authorities that birth defects have risen dramatically in recent years.) Metabolic disease can result from injury or other trauma and are the diseases which do not result from long-term physical degeneration.

Dr. Kelley's experience with over 33,000 benefactors leads him to believe that balancing body chemistry through nutrition is a fruitful approach which should be investigated on a larger scale. How long this investigation will take, or whether it will be done at all are matters of speculation. Many readers or their friends are desperately seeking help for conditions that could be alleviated through nutritional balancing of body chemistry. Cancer is just one of these conditions. A large part of Dr. Kelley's Nutritional Counseling is devoted to planning nutritional programs for people who do not have cancer. Whatever the specific metabolic-degenerative condition may be, hope and encouragement are justified by the many favorable reports from those who have already benefited from Metabolic Medicine.

Warning & Disclaimer

Warning of Fraud

From Park Avenue in New York City to the Motel Clinics and marble palaces of Northern Mexico, from doctors who claim to be medical shcool graduates to those who have bought mail-order diplomas, from the local fly-by-night promoters to the international multi-level conglomerate giants; deception, misrepresentation, and outright fraud is inflicted daily upon a multitude of desperate cancer victims. Orthodox physicians, as well as alternative and complementary health care "doctors" commit plunder, murder and abound in fraud to unprecedented heights never before known to mankind. Many of these unscrupulous individuals claim they are using Dr. Kelley's program or supplements formulated by Dr. Kelley, or an improvement over Dr. Kelley's concepts, etc. None of these wicked, lawless creatures can approach Dr. Kelley's cancer cure success rate. These creatures make false claims that they are using Dr. Kelley's methods and/or have studied with Dr. Kelley. Nothing could be further from the truth. They want you to think their programs are as good or better than Dr. Kelley's Original metabolic Medicine's Cancer Cure Program®. They try to deceive you using Dr. Kelley as an authority figure when they do not even comprehend his concepts.

"Cancer" is Impossible to "Cure"

You can live a long "cancer free" life by following Dr. Kelley's Metabolic Medicine's 'Cancer' paradigm. Dr. Kelley is "cancer free" now and has been since his recovery from terminal pancreatic cancer in 1963. You the "cancer victim" and only you can properly treat your "cancer" by understanding what "cancer" is and following Dr. Kelley's paradigm. Any other procedure is pure fraud, greed and ignorance to the point of stupidity.

The Choice is Up to You

"CANCER CURE" - legally - absence of malignant tumors, malignant blood or lymph abnormalities 5 years after initial biopsy diagnosis. Occurs in 0% to 20% of population using orthodox protocols. Occurs in 4% to 31% of population using alternative medical protocols.

"CANCER CURE" - complete - absence of malignant tumors, malignant blood or lymph abnormalities indefinitely without metabolic support and dietary changes after initial biopsy diagnosis. Occurs in less than 1% of population.

"CANCER FREE" - absence of malignant tumors, malignant blood or lymph abnormalities indefinitely, using metabolic, dietary and detoxification support. Occurs in 93% to 100% of population using Dr. Kelley's metabolic medicine's protocols.

Contents

SECTION I

Cancer Can Be Cured

Chapter One

What is Cancer?

"Cancer" is a term used in error by the medical community to classify a fast-growing malignant tumor, which, if allowed to grow unchecked, will cause death.

Many clinicians have the mistaken belief that cancer is complex; a number of different diseases, each having its own cause. Nothing could be further from the truth.

Most doctors, even research scientists, suppose such things as viruses, X-rays cigarette smoking, chemicals, sunlight, trauma cause cancer. These causes are an indirect stimulation of a normal **TRO-PHOBLAST CELL** into making a false placenta, a malignant tumor mass, and the medical community is in total error in calling them cancer.

In the Beginning

Cancer is the most normal function of one's body. If it were not for cancer, you would not be here. You would not have been born if your mother had not had cancer. Cancer is a normal, necessary metabolic function to form life and continue our species.

Every day every one of us develops cancer – normal cancer cells – Trophoblast Cells. Every day every one of us digests these normal cancer – Trophoblast Cells. We go about the activities of our lives unaware of and oblivious to the cancer process going on within our bodies.

Cancer is a normal, necessary part of life. When your father's sperm invaded your mother's egg, your physical life began. If you grew from that point into an embryo, you would not live – you would fall out of your mother's uterus.

Yahweh, God Almighty, in his wisdom has assured the continuation of our human species by establishing two cycles of physical life – Asexual Generation and Sexual Generation.

The asexual part of life The fertilized egg, properly called the Zygote, forms the Trophoblast which forms the "primitive" germ-cell – this "primitive" germ cell grows and divides by doubling many times into many potential humans – the primary germ-cells.

The sexual part of life: One of the primary germ cells forms the embryo – the remaining primary germ cells start their journey throughout the somatic cell mass (normal body cells) to collect in the testes or the ovaries, waiting to form the next generation of the species. About one-third of these primary germ cells, traveling within the embryonic body cells toward the testes and ovaries, come to occupy all sorts of abnormal positions within one's body.

When the primary germ cells that did not make it to the testes and ovaries, being trapped within normal body tissue, are stimulated, they start to grow and reproduce. The Trophoblast cells (cancer cells) now trapped outside of the uterus, grow rapidly, trying to form a placenta (a malignant tumor mass); this happens in every one of us every day.

The trophoblast cells grow rapidly and uncontrollably, having the ability to invade (metastasize) the wall of your mother's uterus to form the cancer mass (placenta). This cancer mass first opens a blood

3

supply to the embryo for nourishment and second, firmly attaches (metastasizes) the placenta (with its blood supply to the walls of the uterus) to protect the embryo from falling out of the uterus – aborting.

A Bonnie Scottish Lassie

For well over a century, it was common talk among the peasant girls of Scotland that should one find a lump (cancer growth) in the breast, she should get pregnant as soon as possible. When these girls lived beyond their reproductive age, their cancer returned and they died. Both these peasants and girls of today have a multitude of tricks in their bag to become pregnant, everything from baking a cake to tripping a boy in the meadow. This "old wives' tale" intrigued the eminent embryologist, John Beard, a professor at Edinburgh University. Beard was a true scientist. It was he who determined what cancer is, how it is formed, why it is formed and how to properly treat it. Some 50 years later Dr. William Donald Kelley, having never heard of Professor Beard, came to the same scientific paradigm. The medical community refuses to accept Dr. Kelley's paradigm, an unfortunate refusal for the thousands who could be properly treated and cured. Dr. Kelley often states, "That's the way it is!" God may bring this truth to the attention of another scientist, years after Kelley's death.

Direct Cause of Cancer

The direct cause of cancer, according to our research, is the changing of an ectopic primary germ cell into an ectopic trophoblast cell. An excess of female sex hormones brings about this change. Both men and women have male and female sex hormones. When this delicate male-female sex hormone balance is upset, cancer may start.

To explain further: In the human life cycle the male sperm unites with the female egg. If this fertilized egg would grow directly into a new baby, we would have no cancer or cancer problems, but nature does not act so simply and directly, for if she did, the newly formed embryo (baby) would fall out of the uterus. Therefore, nature had to develop some way to attach the new embryo to the wall of the uterus and some way to nourish (feed) it.

After the sperm in the fallopian tube of the mother fertilizes the egg, the fertilized egg gives rise to four basic kinds of cells:

Trophoblast cells which form:

Primitive germ cells, which form:

Primary germ cells, one of which forms the embryo, which form:

Normal body or somatic cells:

Many Primary germ cells which migrate to the testes or ovaries waiting to form the next generation. Many are trapped within the normal body cells and come to occupy all sorts of abnormal positions within the new embryo's body and upon stimulation by female hormones;

Trophoblast cells that form:

A placenta in any place of the embryo's body as it grows to a child or adult.

These out-of-place placentas are, in error, called by the medical community **CANCER.**

By the third day, the fertilized egg has fallen into the uterus. During those three days and for many days thereafter the trophoblast cells (cancer cells) grow rapidly and surround the other two types of cells (primitive germ cells and normal body or somatic cells).

The new baby will fall out of the uterus unless something happens fast, and happen it does. The trophoblast cells metastasize (as cancer does) to the wall of the uterus. Now the baby cannot fall out of the mother's uterus, but needs nourishment. The trophoblast cells (cancer cells) continue to grow rapidly and form the placenta. Now with a good food supply and no danger of falling out of the mother, the baby (embryo) can continue to grow, safe and sound, until birth.

The placental trophoblast tissue (cancer mass) continues to grow until about the seventh week when the baby's pancreas develops. The baby's pancreatic enzyme production along with the mother's pancreatic enzyme production stops the growth of the placental trophoblastic tissue (cancer mass). As the new embryo (baby) is being formed from the normal body or somatic cells, the primary germ cells (pre-placenta cells) are multiplying. In a few days, when the embryo (baby) develops to the proper stage, the primary germ cells stop multiplying and begin to migrate to the gonads (ovaries or testes).

About three billion of these primary germ cells fatigue and never have the vital force necessary to reach the gonads. This means that there are two germ cells for evey area the size of a pinhead dispesed throughout your body. Any one of these germ cells is a potential malignant tumor mass (cancer). That is why a malignant tumor mass (cancer) can form in any part of the body. All that is needed to create a malignant tumor mass in our body is a deficiency of pancreatic enzymes, an imbalance of sex hormones and the embryonic destiny of these primary germ cells to form trophoblast cells, which then forms a false placenta (a malignant tumor) in preparation for the creation of a baby. The imbalance of sex hormones can take place at any time, but usually occurs between 45 and 60 years of age.

When all is said and done, a malignant tumor mass (cancer) is a normal growth of tissue (a placenta) due to the development of a basic (primary) germ cell in the wrong place (outside of the uterus). Sometimes this placenta also has a "baby" or begins a tumor inside of it much like a normal pregnancy — only it is in the wrong place. (When dissecting tumors pathologists often find partially formed teeth, toenails and other types of tissue, such as lung tissue, within the malignant tumor masses.

Malignancy, therefore, is never normal (somatic) tissue gone into wild proliferation, but a normal primary germ cell growing normally in the wrong place.

Physiology of Cancer

I would like to share with you my concept of the physiology of cancer. In order for you to comprehend my concept let me give you a little background by reviewing with you pellagra and diabetes.

Pellagra Can Be Controlled

For years patients were placed in insane asylums because they had the simple deficiency disease called pellagra. In 1916 Dr. Joseph Goldberger found that diet could control or prevent this condition, but it was not until the 1940's that it was discovered the pellagra was nothing more than a simple B vitamin deficiency. Now no knowledgeable physician would commit such a patient, but rather give him B vitamins

What is pellagra? It is a symptom of a general systemic condition. For centuries only the symptoms were treated — now we know better.

Diabetes Can Be Controlled

What is diabetes? It is nothing more than a symptom, a symptom that tells us that our systemic carbohydrate (sugar) metabolism is not functioning properly.

Before the discovery of insulin by professor Ernest L. Scott in 1911 and until the early 1930's, when a person was diagnosed as having diabetes, they would often ask the doctor if their condition could be helped or made worse by what they were eating and should they change their diet in any way. The doctor would tell them: "Oh no, diet doesn't make any difference — eat anything you want, you aren't going to live much longer anyway, so live it up and eat whatever you want." Doctors could not connect the diet and diabetes. Even lay people in those days figured out that if you ate a lot of leafy green vegetables and reduced the amount of sugar you took in, you survived longer and did well — at least better than persons who did not watch their diet.

And so it was that after the development of insulin, doctors figured out that there *is* a factor in diet. In the early 1920s there were few analytical facilities available. But the doctors empirically found that the people who ate green leafy vegetables and a few other foods, survived diabetes much better, and the sugar count in their urine was much better. They had a saying in the medical community at that time that leafy, green vegetables contained "natural insulin." It wasn't actually the truth, but they became aware of the fact that including these vegetables in the diet did play a role and they were trying to explain it.

We are in the same situation now with cancer. Someday in the near future it will dawn on the medical community that diet does make quite a difference in people with cancer and greatly affects health in general. It cannot happen too soon, and when it does, a lot of lives will be saved and a lot of lives will be lived more healthfully.

Most Cancers Can Be Controlled and/or Prevented

At least 97% of all cancer conditions could be adequately treated and/or prevented by diet and pancreatic enzymes. Cancer is a symptom of inadequate and deficient protein metabolism. The real problem is protein metabolism, not cancer. Cancer is only a symptom, telling those who would listen that their protein metabolism is in serious trouble. Surgery, radiation or chemotherapy only treat the symptoms of cancer.

One hundred years ago Dr. John Beard of the University of Edinburgh discovered that the body's primary mechanism for destroying cancer is contained in pancreatin, a secretion from the pancreas that includes enzymes for digesting protein (among other things). Enzymes digest or liquefy foods for absorption by the body. Dr. Beard presented pictures in his books and papers to show recoveries using pancreatin. This was an unprecedented approach to treating the symptoms of cancer — a direct attack on the malignancy with a substance that did not have toxic side effects on the other functions of the body.

Dr. Howard Beard (no relation), a retired Yale University Professor, of Fort Worth, Texas contributed considerably to the understanding and use of pancreatic enzymes in the treatment of cancer. He and other researchers indicated that where cancer is concerned, trypsin and particularly chymotrypsin are the important enzymes in pancreatin. Dr. Beard also recommended a nutritional program and other things, as stated in his book: *A New Approach to Cancer, Rheumatic, and Heart Diseases.*

Cancer Compared to Diabetes

- Diabetes is a disorder of carbohydrate metabolism due to inadequate production or utilization of insulin. Cancer is a disorder of protein metabolism due to inadequate production or utilization of protein digesting enzymes.
- Insulin is produced in the pancreas. Protein-digesting enzymes are produced in the pancreas.
- A neurological process controls insulin production. A neurological process controls enzyme production.
- Diabetes can often be controlled by diet alone. Cancer can often be controlled by diet alone.
- Diabetes can almost always be controlled by the proper dosage of insulin. Cancer can almost always be controlled by proper dosage of protein-digesting enzymes.
- A diabetic patient can live a long useful life and never die as the result of diabetes. A cancer patient can live a long and useful life and never die as the result of cancer.
- Diabetic patients must control their diabetes the rest of their lives by diet or medication or a combination of both. Cancer patients must control their cancer the rest of their lives by diet and protein-digesting enzymes.
- Diabetic patients and cancer patients alike must seek professional help to determine and regulate the condition, but it is up to the individual to administer to the proper diet and missing medication and/or supplements.

Four Laws of Cancer

You cannot have cancer unless three factors are present:

1. The Presence of an ectopic germ cell
2. The Stimulating presence of the female sex hormones
3. A Deficiency of active pancreatic enzymes

First Law: Body Fails to Produce Adequate Amount of Active Pancreatic Enzymes for One of Three Reasons:

- 83% — Overworking the pancreas by the intake of too much protein
- 10% — Neurological injury to pancreatic enzyme production
- 7% — Malfunction of body chemistry inactivating the enzymes

Second Law: Protein Is Gradually Sapped from Muscles

Our research indicates that in 93% of all cancer cases the development of cancer is gradual. The average cancer patient has had cancer 39 months before it is clinically diagnosed. The important factor here is **not** that it is slow-growing, but rather what happens to the body during this growth time. The body must have protein to live, but during these 39 months, the body could not get enough protein from its food supply. Therefore, to keep the blood protein at a minimal level to sustain life, the body gradually saps or destroys the muscles of the body.

Third Law: Damaged Tissue and Female Hormones at the Site of a Latent, Misplaced Ectopic Germ Cell Set the Scene for Cancer

At this point the conditions are ripe for the symptom cancer to develop. All that is needed is something to stimulate the female sex hormone formation at the site of a misplaced ectopic germ cell. This simulation is most often done by scar formation caused by a blow, bruise, drop of tar in the lung, sunburn, overdose of X-ray, or anything else that can cause a normal scar formation procedure to take place in the body — at the site of a latent ectopic germ cell. This is normal wear and tear of the body, which happens to each of us every day; it is only when our protein metabolism is deficient that the symptom cancer develops.

Now the ectopic germ cell mistakenly thinks it is time to have a baby and starts growing a placenta (cancer) in preparation for a baby that never develops. The only trouble is, without proper amounts of pancreatic enzymes circulating in our bloodstream to dissolve this abnormal placenta, it keeps growing and does not stop. When the patient finally consults the physician, the condition of cancer is announced and surgery, radiation and/or chemotherapy are recommended.

Fourth Law: For Cancer to Be Cured There Must Be Positive Change in the Physiology of the Patient

If nothing changes in the physiology of the patient, the cancer grows until it destroys the body. If positive changes occur in the physiology of the patient one of two things can happen:

- One person with cancer lasts a long time while another person with the same type of cancer goes rapidly — and, before now, no one knew why.
- The right combination of circumstances occurs, and the cancer is dissolved or "cured."

This book answers the question: "What is the right combination of circumstances?"

Metabolic Medicine's Cancer Cure Program

"Metabolic" pertains to metabolism: The chemical and physical processes continuously going on in living organisms and cells, comprising those by which assimilated food is built up (anabolism) into protoplasm and those by which protoplasm is used and broken down (catabolism) into simpler substances or waste matter, with the release of energy for all vital processes.

The person who has the metabolic malfunction should be addressed, not the disease that has the person. We call our system of addressing cancer "Metabolic" because the total person and all of his chemical and physical processes must be considered and new habits of health developed in order to obtain a reasonable state of health.

We advise a comprehensive program, extremely effective and inexpensive when compared to surgery, radiation and/or chemotherapy. Those willing to faithfully and tediously follow the program will be successful and those who follow it in part or haphazardly will be completely unsuccessful.

Metabolic Medicine's Cancer Cure Program® is based on the best scientific knowledge available and has been condensed to a simple, well-balanced system. Metabolic Medicine's Cancer Cure Program® can be compared to a fine watch; each part must be there and working properly or it does not work at all. Each step of Metabolic Medicine's Cancer Cure Program® must be followed exactly or there will be no relief of the symptoms.

Five Steps of Metabolic Medicine's Cancer Cure Program:

1. Metabolic Supplementation (Chapter Three)

2. Detoxification of the Body (Chapter Four)

3. Adequate, Proper, Well-Balanced Diet (Chapter Five)

4. Neurological Stimulation (Chapter Six)

5. Spiritual Attitude (Chapter Seven)

1.   Halting or stopping the malignant growth with the use of supplemental metabolic nutrition, is relatively simple. The growth is usually stopped from within 3 hours to 3 weeks of metabolic nutritional supplementation, depending upon the amount and method of administration. This is usually noted by a sharp elevation of body temperature lasting about three days.

2.   The clinical problem in treating a cancer patient is clearing the body of accumulated toxins, growth stoppage, takes from 3 weeks to 12 months, depending upon the location and mass (amount) of growth. Many cancer patients have had their tumors successfully treated only to die of toxic poisons as

the mass is dissolved and excreted from the body — in a case such as this the clinician treated the disease and not the patient or failed to treat "metabolically."

3.   Diet for the cancer victim is as important as diet for the diabetic, and should be carefully followed during the first year of the recovery process. Later, diet can be altered to a more acceptable protocol. However, for the rest of one's life food intake and enzymes must be considered to remain "cancer-free."

4.   The nerve pathways to the pancreas must remain functional, turning the pancreas on and off as needed. When this process fails, the pancreas does not know what to do. Osteopathic and chiropractic adjustments, as well as acupuncture and other newer neurological therapies have also proven helpful to the cancer victim.

5.   Spiritual attitude often means the difference between life and death. Many are not dedicated to the hard work and faith required for success. One patient recovered by renting funny movies like Abbot and Costello, the Marx Brothers, Charlie Chapman and other noted comedians. He literally laughed himself well.

We find that the rate of recovery is subject to another law — that of blood supply. If the rate of blood supply to an area is great, recovery is fast. If the blood supply to an area is inadequate, recovery is slow. Thus, we find those with leukemia respond quickly, while those with bone afflictions have a much slower response. We have also noted that in tumors of large diameter (three or more inches) the outside diameter is quickly dissolved, but the interior, where there is a lack of blood supply, often takes several months to dissolve. This slow response is a wonderful thing: The body has time to detoxify and the death rate from toxemia is greatly reduced.

The prognosis for a cancer patient is good when the liver, kidney, and lung functions are at least 50% of normal, and an optimistic spiritual attitude is maintained. Unfortunately, we have found many people who have lost hope, or their next of kin have lost hope, to the degree they were resigned to death and refused to try our Cancer Cure Program.

Metabolic Cancer Defense

There are only two Physicians — the Almighty and your own body

The pancreas is a complex organ with many functions and purposes. Briefly mentioned here are three:

A. Carbohydrate (Sugar) Metabolism.

If this pancreatic function fails, the resulting disease process is what we call diabetes.

B.   Production of Digestive Enzymes:

- **Amylase**, which digests starches, glycogen and other carbohydrates.
- **Lipase**, which digests fats.
- **Protease**, which digests proteins. If this pancreatic function fails, the resulting disease process is called:

    a.   Cystic Fibrosis (usually in children) and/or;

    b.   Malnutrition, starvation, cachexia, wasting, or emaciation (usually in adults).

C. To Digest or Cannibalize:

- Intercellular metabolic waste and toxic metabolic materials.

- Intracellular waste products and dead or dysfunctional normal cells.
- Normal dormant pre-placenta cells as they become cancer cells.

When this pancreatic function fails, we have the resulting disease process we call cancer.

Metabolic Ignorance

Many causes exist for the failure of the pancreatic metabolic function. Often more than one cause exists simultaneously within the cancer patient. Listed below are some of these causes and all must be considered as possible or ruled out as non-causative in each cancer patient:

- **The pancreas** fails to produce an adequate quantity of enzymes.
- **We take** into our bodies such large quantities of foods, which require pancreatic enzymes for their digestion, that there are no enzymes available for cancer digestion.
- **Diet:** Incorrect type, amount, and timing of nutritional intake.
- **Nutritional Components** are not available (vitamins, minerals, amino acids, etc.) that are necessary for normal metabolism within the pancreas.
- **We may fail** to take into our diet enough minerals, which are essential to release the enzymes into activity.
- **We may produce** enough enzymes but fail to take into our diet enough coenzymes (vitamins) to make the enzymes work.
- **Obstruction** of pancreatic secretion flow.
- **Often** we produce enough enzymes, but the blood supply to a cancer area is so poor, the enzymes we produce are not carried to the area.
- **Proper pH Balance** (acid/alkaline balance) within the intestinal tract and/or within the cancer tumor mass.
- **Infection:** Bacterial or viral.
- **Chemical Poisons** within the patient's body from the environment, food chain, drugs, metabolic wastes or medications.
- **Man-Made Biologicals**: Viruses or infectious agents.
- **Emotional** instability and/or trauma.
- **Non-Absorption** of pancreatic secretions (pancreatin) from the intestines into the body due to mucus, scarring or damage to the small intestine from various diseases.
- **Our bodies produce** anti-enzyme factors. These factors keep the enzymes from digesting our own bodies. Sometimes we produce an over-abundant supply of these anti-enzyme factors.
- **Balance:** Instability and weakness of the autonomic nervous system.
- **Genetic:** Inheriting a small, weak or defective (ineffective) pancreas.
- **Radiation Damage** such as from therapeutic procedures, etc.
- **Spiritual** weakness.

Racial Gene Pools

The pure white race, Aryans, and in particular, the Anglo-Saxon, Celtic, Scandinavian, Germanic, French, Scottish, Irish and British peoples, genetically appear to have a much higher incidence of cancer than other races. The Jewish race, as well as Blacks, Asians and mixed races have a much lower incidence of cancer than the Aryan race.

Other races have cancer, of course, but in proportion to the pancreatic damage from malnutrition, viruses or infection. In addition, the percentage of cancer within the other races can be correlated to the percentage of white blood mixed in the individual's gene pool.

Cancer Recovery

**All persons who have cancer die of starvation, unless
they are first killed through improper treatment or methods.**

In attempting to find help and in helping others, one must comprehend the four basic parameters one confronts:

First, the stricken cancer victim and their family members have been so deceived by the Establishment that they are completely brainwashed and put in overwhelming fear.

Second, another parameter we often forget is that once a cancer victim or family member has awakened from this imprisoned condition — they trust no one. All too often, the mindset of the cancer victim is to demand an immediate, noticeable, positive, measurable response. When this response is not forthcoming, they usually flip and flounder around, in and out of all forms of therapies claimed by their promoters as "the cure." Usually, most of the individuals who finally find Dr. Kelley's Metabolic Medicine's Cancer Cure Program® are these disappointed and disillusioned persons; without hope and adequate funding for recovery. Such persons must have at least 6 months of life and follow the Metabolic Program most carefully. Then, if they survive that long, there is a excellent chance of recovery. This recovery period is a long and tedious one, usually lasting at least 2 years. After that, they must take a form of metabolic support for the rest of their lives.

Third, most of these individuals expect and demand immediate results or they go on to other therapies. This, however, is not the way one recovers from cancer. It is not the way they developed cancer.

It requires the failure of the pancreas from 2 to 4 years to develop a malignant tumor mass — which the medical community in error calls "cancer."

It requires at least the same length of time to clean up a ravaged body. Then the process of rebuilding the body can take place, which usually takes an additional 2 to 4 years of hard work and living right. Then, for the rest of one's life, one must keep a constant vigil to remain free of malignant tumor masses.

Fourth, one must realize that physicians are forbidden to treat CANCER. The controlled medical Establishment has several methods and techniques to prohibit a physician from treating cancer.

Physicians are only allowed to treat malignant tumor masses.

Dr. Morrision and I have experienced most of these diabolical acts of injustice, not only to the cancer victim, but also to the physician.

Cancer: A "Process" Not An "Object"

Daily, everyone produces malignant tumor cells and daily, most everyone's pancreas produces adequate pancreatin to digest the food they eat and these malignant tumor cells. **When one's pancreas fails to produce the necessary pancreatin to accomplish these tasks, a disease "process" takes place which we correctly call cancer.**

When this disease process occurs, people are not aware of it. As it is so subtle it must progress for 2 to 4 years before physicians realize they are in trouble. The things people often complain about to their physician during this time are indigestion and weight loss at first then, a few months later, excessive weight gain, eye trouble and pyorrhea. Eventually a large enough malignant tumor mass forms — which is the "object" or result of the disease process that we correctly call cancer — that the cancer victim and their physicians can observe and in error call **cancer.**

The objective of Metabolic Medicine's Cancer Cure Program is to supply the body with adequate pancreatin to properly digest food, stop this disease process and to rid the body of any and all malignant tumor masses. This is the proper, normal, physiological method of taking care of the disease process we correctly call **cancer.**

Cancer Markers

Pancreatin digests the malignant tumor masses and cells into liquid debris. This debris is then gobbled up by the white blood cells and removed from the body by way of bile from the liver, which goes into the colon and out, and urine from the kidneys, which goes into the bladder and out. A small amount of this debris leaves the body by way of skin perspiration as well as hair and nail growth.

Upon starting Metabolic Medicine's Cancer Cure Program, two measurable things occur:
- White blood cells increase in number, which is considered by everyone to be a good sign.
- Cancer markers become temporarily elevated, which often scares both cancer victims and their doctors. Dr. Kelley considers elevated cancer markers to be a good sign for the following reason:

The malignant tumor mass debris consists, in part, of cancer marker components. Until now most of this cancer marker material has been held in the tissue surrounding the malignant tumor mass and usually increases when masses continue to develop. Upon starting Metabolic Medicine's Cancer Cure Program the cancer markers are released into the bloodstream as the masses are digested, causing a high volume of cancer marker material to appear in the bloodstream temporarily and is the most misinterpreted part of the Metabolic Medicine's Cancer Cure Program®. The second most misinterpreted part is that often the malignant tumor masses continue to grow temporarily before one's normal metabolic function can take over.

Why You Will Feel Bad During Recovery

When the organs of detoxification become overloaded with debris, one feels lousy — like you were run over by a freight train (see page 75). This lousy feeling is how you will know that Dr. Kelley's Metabolic Medicine's Program is working.

If you do not feel lousy one of two things is happening:

- You are not taking enough pancreatin of the correct quality or quantity
- You have a very small amount of malignant tumor cells and/or masses

We expect all cancer victims taking pancreatin to feel toxic (sore, headachy, no energy, nauseous, irritable, elevated temperature, flu-like symptoms, etc.). Occurrence of these symptoms indicates one's metabolic functions are working well. At this time we recommend that you stop taking the Metabolic Nutrients for 5 days to allow your organs of detoxification time to remove this debris from your body.

Many cancer victims have only a small malignant tumor mass and experience only mild discomfort while other cancer victims have large malignant tumor masses like the actor Steve McQueen (see page 125). If your physician surgically removes most of such masses, your recovery time speeds up.

Reactions while on the Kelley Program

Reactions and Notes

We have found that on occassion an area of a malignant tumor mass becomes tender and swells. This could be a very good sign. As one's body cleans up the various debris and digested cells, it is like hitting your finger with a hammer - tenderness, pain and swelling occur. Also very frightening to some who have a tingling or "electrical shock" sensation. This is usually caused by pressure on nerves from Malignant tumor growth placing pressure. But often it also occurs when the swelling from clean-up going on within the body. Therefore, it could be a good or a bad sign, but one should consider the good possibility of clean-up activity.

Once or twice after some months on our Metabolic Program, a family member has called me and said, "your program didn't work" Bob/Mary died. When questioned, the individual had not been on the program for the last four to six months. Another time a call came in saying the individual had died, only to find out she was killed instantly in a head-on auto accident. Others have died from gunshot wounds while dear hunting. Others from heart attacks. Of course, this is not a Metabolic failure.

World War III

We have been plunged into World War III by our Common Enemy. The major dilemma we are encountering is that we, you and I, do not recognize that we are in the middle of World War III - let alone who **is our enemy**. No metabolic program will keep you well and healthy when you are subject to being attacked by biological warfare agents via Chem-trails, vaccinations, drugs, contaminated food and water.

Chapter Two

Do I Have Cancer?

Have you ever asked yourself this question?

If our nation can put a man on the moon and place a satellite in orbit for the banks and stock markets to transfer money and assets out of the country — tax free — why has the cure for cancer not been found?

It has!

Biopsy

For years patients were placed in insane asylums because they had the simple deficiency disease called pellagra. In 1916, Dr. Joseph Goldberger found that diet could prevent this condition, but it was not until the 1940's that it was discovered that pellagra was nothing more than a simple B vitamin deficiency. Now no knowledgeable physician would commit such a patient, but rather give him B vitamins. What is pellagra? It is a symptom of a general systemic condition. For centuries only the symptoms were treated – now we know better.

The only accepted legal medical diagnosis of cancer is by biopsy. This is not 100% accurate, for there are false positives as well as false negative biopsies. We, that is you and I, are neither permitted to make a diagnosis of cancer nor by law to use any system of diagnosis except biopsy for cancer diagnosis. The medical Establishment tightly controls the diagnosis of cancer.

Everybody Has Cancer

Each day each one of us has a "cancer" start and develop in our body, a normal ongoing process each one of us experiences. Usually, our normal metabolic defense system takes care of these wayward cancer cells and we go about our daily lives unaware that any of this is taking place. It is when our normal metabolic defense system or clean-up crew cannot handle this normal body process that we begin to develop a tumor or mass which can eventually be found by ourselves or our physician. Before this happens, you can easily determine the failure of your defense system and the beginning of "cancer" — Malignant Tumor Masses — by using the following simple pancreas self-examination.

Dr. Kelley's Self-examination Procedure

There are only three who care about you: God, yourself and sometimes your mother.

The Establishment has finally come to strongly encourage all of us to practice self-examination for cancer. Women are told to examine their breasts once a month. All of us are told to carefully examine for lumps, bumps and skin changes to help us become aware of our body and seek medical care early if needed. We have had, from the first publication of this book in 1967, the self-examination for the earliest possible development of pancreatic malfunction. When this occurs, within 2 to 4 years one always develops a malignant tumor mass, which the medical community, in error, labels cancer.

You give yourself control with Dr. Kelley's Self-Examination Procedure of one's pancreas. If one finds a pancreatic malfunction in time to properly treat it, one will have to do it for one's self. Dr. Kelley's Self-Examination of one's pancreas finds pancreas malfunction long before malignant tumor masses form. You have the greatest to gain by self-examination. God gives one the intelligence and self will to do this if one's mother, family or friends do not interfere.

The Self-Examination Procedure outlined below should be the most important part of your health program. This procedure only indicates the activity of one's pancreas — it is not a diagnostic test. It only alerts one very early to the possible formation of malignant tumor masses. Thus, you can go to your physician for proper and legal diagnosis and treatment if needed. This procedure is the most sensitive and early awareness system known to date.

Dr. Kelley's Self-Examination Procedure is nothing more than early self-detection and/or an early warning of the decrease of pancreatic production of adequate pancreatic enzymes.

When the pancreas is not working properly and fails to produce adequate amounts of enzymes the following occurs:

- Indigestion with belching and passing of excessive gas (flatulence).
- Over an extended time, the dental condition called pyorrhea.
- Focusing problems of the eyes. This occurs because the muscles of the eyes are so tiny it takes little protein loss to interfere with their function; a tiny little bit of eye muscle makes a big difference. (Dr. Kelley is still able to read without glasses at the age of 75—and uses the same pair of glasses to drive as he used in 1963. See his story, "38-Year Victory Over Pancreatic/Liver Cancer" on page 109.)

Dr. Kelley correctly calls such conditions pancreatic failure, and within two to four years normal trophoblast cells (false placenta cells) produced by the trapped primary germ cells will develop into malignant tumor masses or lymph and blood dysfunction.

As stated elsewhere in this book, the disease commonly referred to as "cancer" by the medical community is nothing more than the failure of one's pancreas to produce adequate enzymes to properly digest one's food intake and cleanup the defective, worn-out and dead cells throughout one's body.

Do-It-Yourself Pancreas Self-examination

It is our belief that each of us has the right to build and maintain a healthy body, mind and spirit by properly addressing pancreas failure by taking adequate, effective pancreatic enzyme supplements by mouth as outlined in Chapter III.

Dr. Kelley's Pancreas Self-Examination below should be the most important part of your cancer prevention regime. This Pancreas Self-Examination only indicates the function or "failure-to-function-properly" of one's pancreas. This procedure is the most sensitive evaluation and early awareness system known to date. It determines the status, condition and activity of one's pancreatic enzyme production. Dr. Kelley's Pancreas Self-Examination Procedure should be done every 12 to 18 months.

Dr. Kelley's Pancreas Self-examination Procedure

Take 6 Formula T capsules with each meal and at bedtime.

Impression of Effects

• If within eight weeks on the Pancreas Self-examination one becomes toxic, ill, crabby, sick, nauseated, vomits, or develops an elevation of temperature or violent headache, a malignant tumor mass of placenta cells could possibly be present of a size that should be detectable by one's physician.

• If within eight weeks on the Pancreas Self-Examination one feels better, has better digestion, more energy and stamina, one is usually pre-cancerous. That is, one's pancreas is not quite able to meet the demands of digestion and the normal clean-up activity needs of one's body. In this case, it is highly likely one will develop a malignant placenta tumor mass within 2 to 4 years.

• If one is pre-cancerous it is suggested one should take two or three Formula Mg capsules with meals and at bedtime the rest of one's life.

• If, after eight weeks on the Pancreas Self-Examination one neither notices a toxic feeling or condition nor does not feel better, one's pancreas is probably producing adequate pancreatic enzymes and it is unlikely a malignant placenta tumor mass is forming. One should repeat the Pancreas Self-Test again every 12 to 18 months.

• There could be a false positive or false negative indication, but this is most rare.

Metabolic Classification of Cancer

Dr. Kelley has classified malignant conditions according the physiology and metabolism of the tissue in which the trapped primary germ cells develop their trophoblast cells begin their aggressive development to form a placenta. In addressing individuals with more than one malignant class, one should support Class I malignancies first before addressing Class II and Class III. Most oncologists treat the most aggressive class first which often resolves the other classes.

Classification of Malignant Tumors

   1. **Class I Malignancies — AIDS**
   2. **Class II Malignancies — Soft tumors, such as Hodgkin's, Leukemia, Lymphoma, Multiple Myeloma, etc.**
   3. **Class III Malignancies — Hard tumors, such as brain, breast, lung, colon, prostate, liver, pancreas, etc.**

Protocol of metabolic support for each of these classes are given in detail in Chapter III.

Life-threatening Crises

By the time one's body forms a malignant placenta tumor mass, which is in error called cancer, one becomes frightened. One's physician also becomes frightened and is only permitted three choices to address the malignant placenta tumor mass, surgery, radiation or chemotherapy. Addressing these malignant placenta tumor masses is absolutely necessary in most cases. However, if one does not properly address the *cause* of one's "cancer," these and other malignant placenta tumor masses will return in a few months even larger, more vicious and life-threatening.

Before, during and after your physician treats these malignant placenta tumor masses, one should address the cause of the cancer — that is, the failure of the pancreas. As outlined in Chapter III, metabolically supporting the failing pancreas is absolutely necessary to properly address the cancer and help prevent the reoccurrence of additional malignant placenta tumor masses.

Invest in Prevention

Prevention is the smart way to go. Protecting your investment, your own body, is the intelligent procedure to best ensure that you never receive a diagnosis of cancer. College of Metabolic Medicine's Formula Mg™ is the best way to survive the insults, stresses, and strains of our lifestyles.

Jesus Christ said, "Physician, Heal Thyself." What is the true teaching behind this beautiful saying? What was Jesus really trying to say? It involves the true meaning of cure — cure for anything. It is often said. "I went to Dr. Jones and he cured me." Nothing could be further from the truth. No matter how many years doctors have gone to school, no matter how many college degrees they may have, doctors can cure only one person — themselves. It is important that you understand that only you can cure you of anything.

It is you and your body chemistry that cures you of your disease. In following this cure, take note that you are environmental, physical, mental and spiritual — each facet plays a part in your "cure." Your physician or clinician can only bring to your attention some of the basic laws of God concerning health. Unfortunately not all clinicians know the laws of God concerning health, even though they are honest and sincere and try their hardest.

Can I Trust My Doctor?

- The answer is a simple, **Yes.**
- **Yes,** you will need all the professional help you can obtain from the medical community.
- **Yes,** you must have help in all the crisis situations you will encounter on the road to health.
- **Yes,** you are required by law to submit to their advice and cooperate in doing the recommendations made.
- **Yes,** your only chance of survival in your battle in this war is to work with your physician.
- **Yes,** but there are many things that are helpful in your fight that your physician cannot do for you. In dealing with your metabolism, you must do it yourself. This book is to help guide you through the things you can do to help yourself and accomplish the best possible state of health.
- **Yes,** work with your physician and do all he or she advised, and study and glean all you can from this book.

Seek A Physician to Work with You, Not on You

Dr. Carol Morrison

My fellow-researcher, Dr. Carol A. Morrison, M.D., F.A.C.C. (Associate Professor, School of Medicine, The University of Pennsylvania for 12 years; ABIM Certified Diplomat in Internal Medicine; ABIM Certified Diplomat Cardiovascular Disease; Diplomat of National Board of Medical Examiners) and I spent 10 years in undivided attention to bring the truth to you: We reviewed thousands of medical records of cancer patients; spent hundreds of hours in Medical School Libraries; we spent thousands of hours in university law libraries; we brought many legal cases into the State and Federal Courts of Pennsylvania; we appealed to the 3rd Circuit of the Federal Courts several times and appealed to the U.S. Supreme Court five times; collected more than adequate data and endured sufficient experiences to be honest and deal with Christian love for our-fellow cancer patients in this book. Without rancor we make the following statements. To put it candidly, we know whereof we speak and write. (See below and take note in chapter ten.)

Dr. Morrison and I were desperately working within the legal system and medical Establishment to be permitted to use Metabolic Medicine's Cancer Cure® to help those who chose to use this proven therapeutic procedure. For years, the medical Establishment, without investigation, said "It couldn't be a 'cancer cure'; Dr. Kelley is a dentist."

Dr. Morrison was of a different mind. She is one of the most outstanding physicians in the United States, Board Certified in Cardiology and Internal Medicine, has taken advanced training with Queen Elizabeth's Physicians and taught at the University of Pennsylvania Medical School.

I know our opinions about the medical Establishment are repulsive and unbelievable to the honest, God-fearing, Christian citizen. Nevertheless, these opinions are true. We have encountered so many such experiences, we must bring to your attention at least one of these horror stories.

Dr. Morrison's Brother David

One day, Dr. Morrison got an urgent call from her brother, David. He had a small lump about the size of a pea, on the left side of his neck, just above the collarbone. His doctor in New Jersey, knowing the stress David was under with his "wife-to-be" told him to calm down, get his family situation resolved, watch the lump and check again in six months. Hearing this advice, David's mother went into hysterics and brought David to Pittsburgh, where Carol was working in a local hospital. Their mother was somewhat justified as both David's father and Carol had been diagnosed by biopsy as having cancer (lung and breast).

Carol knew from her medical training that if the lump was malignant, it was only a metastasis of a tumor mass, usually found in the chest between the lungs. She asked me to ask the Holy Spirit for confirmation. I was told that, yes, the original malignant mass had been between the lungs, but the normal body defenses (clean-up crew) had completely cleared the primary site, the lump in the neck had been encapsulated into a fibrous nodule, and he should leave it alone and get David's love life settled to reduce his stress — the same advice his New Jersey doctor had given. To verify the Holy Spirit, Carol did a "scan" in the hospital where she was working; it was negative.

It was agreed to wait six months and then check David again. David's mother, wanting to play doctor as many unqualified people do, took David to Philadelphia to the medical school at the University of Pennsylvania. She demanded the nodule be removed and biopsied to prove it was cancer.

A rich mother and David's health insurance policy was like waving a red flag in front of a bull. If she demanded a diagnosis of cancer and could pay for it, "she will get it." And David was fair game to the medical con artists.

Second Opinion

Second Opinion Time: If you are rich enough and live on the East Coast, it's Memorial Sloan-Kettering Cancer Center in New York City; if you are rich enough and live in Texas, it's M.D. Anderson Cancer Center in Houston. If you are rich enough and live in the central U.S., it's The Mayo Clinic in Rochester, Minnesota. If you are rich enough and live on the West Coast, it's Stanford in California. Everyone gets a piece of the pie!

The advice of the New York doctors was: "The University of Pennsylvania uses exactly the same therapy as we do and could treat David as well as we do. We do see a swelling in the nasal sinus. It would be closer to home for David to be treated in Philadelphia and less stress."

Back in Philadelphia mother demanded a biopsy of the nasal sinus; the fact that David had allergies was never considered. The surgery was a disaster. The surgeon ruptured a major artery and nearly killed David. No biopsy of a life-or-death situation was encountered. All manner of chemotherapy and radiation was then started.

Third Opinion

David's mother heard (through the patient's gossip hotline) of the newest procedure in Pittsburgh and announced: "We must have this 'newest and best' for David." She loved to play doctor.

In Pittsburgh David was scalped: His skull was sawed from ear to ear and set aside. Seventeen biopsy samples were taken, digging as close to the brain as possible. His skull was replaced and his scalp sewn back over the bones: Seventeen hours and $200,000 later David was wheeled out of the operating room.

David was seeing five doctors and each was giving him something different and not knowing or caring what the others were treating him with. All this was accomplished and treatment performed when there was no positive biopsy ever reported. All they could say was: "It could be cancer, but we can't find it in the biopsy." Mother was delighted; she got to play doctor along with the best of them, while being relieved of part of her wealth.

Dr. Morrison and I were devastated. We constantly asked God why such devastating and cruel experiences were necessary *when David did not even have cancer!* Maybe it was for you, the readers of this book — for your education and understanding. Carol and I had seen enough, long before David.

David's Death

As a result of the best of the orthodox medical community, his physicians, who inflicted surgery, radiation and chemotherapy upon him, murdered David. Such forms of murder are socially accepted, standard acceptable procedure in treating cancer victims.

Chapter Three

Metabolic Supplementation

Cancer is basically a deficiency disease — a deficiency of the pancreatic enzymes, a deficiency of the free active enzymes in the tissues of the body.

The 1994 Hatch Act

Since 1994 and the passage of the Hatch Act, individuals and physicians may legally support human metabolism by diet, nutritional supplements and certain procedures, as long as they are not harmful. In fact, for many years it has been accepted that one must add vitamins, minerals, trace minerals, amino acids, etc. to the human diet to support and maintain health. We are bombarded daily with the advertising of many "fortified" products that inform us of the necessity of supplying the body's metabolic needs.

Missing Nutrients

The modern diet is quite deficient in certain foods that have in the past been mainstays of good nutrition and the support of health. The most outstanding missing group as a whole is the organ meats, such as kidney, liver, stomach, intestinal tract tripe, and lung. These health-building foods are unheard of and unavailable in today's society; to get these today, one must obtain them in the form of nutritional supplements.

Sweetbreads

Pancreas tissue or sweetbreads without a doubt, indicated by our 30-odd years of research, is the most deficient item in our food chain. It should be noted that the pancreas is the most needed of all the missing organ meats from our diets and must be supplied in our diets or serious deficiencies result.

Low temperature processed pancreas gland enzymes are available to the public in various Metabolic Formulas listed below. These nutritional products are designed to support the normal metabolic processes of human metabolism.

Metabolic Nutritional Supplementation

Below are the Metabolic Formulas Dr. Kelley's counselees have taken and used over the past 38 years. These Formulas have been helpful to thousands of his metabolic counselees.

The College of Metabolic Medicine's products listed below are manufactured to Dr. Kelley's exact specifications and under his direct supervision.

A. Metabolic Formulas A, Ca+, L, and P, Mg, and T

1. **Formula A™**—For those who have been diagnosed by their physician as having Class I Malignancies—AIDS. (For the amount to take and the timing see below.)
2. **Formula Ca+™**—For those who have been diagnosed by their physician as having Class III Malignancies, or tested positive on Dr. Kelley's Pancreas Self-Examination Procedure (see page 17) or those who have been diagnosed by their physician as having cancer. This is a powerful multi-glandular enzyme formulation. (For the amount to take and the timing, see below.)
3. **Formula L™**—For those who have been diagnosed by their physician as having Class II Malignancies, such as leukemia. (For the amount to take and the timing see below.)
4. **Formula Mg™**—For those who have not been diagnosed with cancer, it has proven to be helpful in prevention of cancer, as well as the digestion of food. This is very powerful Multi-Glandular Enzyme Formulation with enzyme activators not only to make it work efficiently, but also to activate one's own pancreatic enzyme production. For prevention, this enzyme formula should be taken with meals (food), two capsules with meals and one with snacks. Formula Mg™ contains enzyme activators lacking in some cancer patients. Formula Mg™ activates the pancreatic juice (peptones) as soon as food from the stomach and peptones from the pancreas arrive in the intestinal tract. A lack of these activators prevents the pancreatic enzymes from digesting food and destroying cancer cells in the body.
5. **Formula P™**—For those who have successfully recovered from cancer, as outlined below, should take three capsules with each meal. Prevention of re-occurrence is this enzyme's contribution to your health. Dr. Kelley takes these daily, "I do not want to have cancer again!"
6. **Formula T™**—Pancreas Self-Examination Test: 6 capsules with each meal and at bedtime (see page 17).

B. Timing of Metabolic Formulas

It is far more important than one can possibly realize to take the Metabolic Formulas at the proper time. The Metabolic Formulas should be taken when the body is in the proper acid/alkaline balance.

A. Ca+ and L should be taken at the following times:

10 Capsules one (1) hour before meals;

12 Capsules with each meal

6 capsules per day taken at bedtime or 3:30 a.m.

Getting Started:

Some have found it easier starting the first week by taking 6 capsules each at the 7 suggested intake times; then 8, then up to the suggested 10/12.

Metabolic Formula Cycles

All metabolic formulas, except Formulas T and Mg, must be cycled on and off. The raw materials for the repair and rebuilding of the body must be cycled. Taking the Metabolic Formulas during the **"On"** cycle provides a saturation of needed nutrients. Stopping the Metabolic Formulas during the **"Off"** cycle provides the necessary time for the body to repair, rebuild and detoxify.

"On" Cycle

Take the Metabolic Formulas for 10 or more days, until one becomes toxic, but no longer than 25 days.

Stop If You Feel Sick

If you become toxic (a 'goopy' sick feeling), ill, nauseated, crabby, have an elevated temperature, or violent headache **Stop** taking the Metabolic Formulas.

It is best to stay **On** your Metabolic Formulas for 10 to 25 days. However, when you suffer negative symptoms anytime after the third day, you may **Stop** taking them at that point.

It is best to continue for 25 days or until toxicity forces you to **Stop.**

"Off" Cycle

Remain **Off** the Metabolic Formulas for 5 days. You must give the body time to detoxify. Stay **Off** the Metabolic Formulas the full 5 days, even if you feel well enough to continue. Give your body time for repair and rebuilding. You must continue your detoxification program during the **"Off"** cycle (See *Chapter Four*).

While "Off" You May Feel Worse

If you feel worse while you are cycling **Off** the Metabolic Formulas it means your body needs them (this is not a toxic reaction), so you should go back **On** them until you feel toxic and try to go **Off** them again in 25 days or when you become toxic.

C. Metabolic Supplementation Support of One's Body

Having Malignant Tumors

*Therapeutic Protocol
A Every 3 hours
3 Niacinamide-B6
2 Cataplex C
B 1 hr. before meals
10 Forumula Ca +
2 Colostrom
2 Pituitary GH Sprays
C Once at Breakfast
1 tbsp. Formula F
2 tbsp. Water of Life
3 RNA
1 Cataplex D
1 Folic Acid B-12
1 tbsp. Magnesium
2 tsp. Selenium
D With each meal
12 Forumula Ca+
2 MSM
3 Adrenal
1 Biost
1 Cal-Ma-Plus
3 Catalyn
1 Co-Q-10
30 drps. Phosfood
2 Cataplex B12
1 tsp. EPN
E At Bedtime/3:30 am
6 Formula Ca+
1 tbsp. Water of Life
2 tsp. Sulfur
1 Pituitary GH Spray
*Take during time of active cancer

*Transition Protocol
A Every 3 hours
2 Niacinamide-B6
2 Cataplex C
B 1 hr. before meals
6 Formula Ca+
2 Colostrom (CHS)
2 Pituitary GH Sprays
C Once at Breakfast
1 tbsp. Formula F
2 tbsp. Water of Life
1 RNA
1 Cataplex D
1 Folic Acid B-12
1 tsp. Magnesium
1 tsp. Selenium
D With each meal
6 Formula Ca+
1 MSM
2 Adrenal
1 Biost
1 Cal-Ma-Plus
3 Catalyn
1 Co-Q-10
30 drps. Phosfood
1 tsp. EPN
1 tbsp. Silver
E At Bedtime/3:30 am
6 Formula Ca+
2 tsp. Water of Life
1 tsp. Sulfur
1 Pituitary GH Spray
*Take for 6 months after being cancer-free

*Maintenance Protocol
A Every 3 hours
2 Niacinamide-B6
2 Cataplex C
B 1 hr. before meals
2 Pituitary GH Sprays

C Once at Breakfast
1 tbsp. Formula F+
2 tbsp. Water of Life
1 RNA
1 Cataplex D
1 tsp. Magnesium
1 tsp. Selenium

D With each meal
3 Forumula Mg
1 MSM
2 Adrenal
1 Biost
1 Cal-Ma-Plus
3 Catalyn
30 drps. Phosfood
1 tsp. EPN
1 Co-Q-10
1 tbsp. Silver
At Bedtime
2 tbsp. Calcium
2 tsp. Water of Life
1 Pituitary GH Spray

*Take for rest of your life

College Health Stores, LLC at 888-477-3618, 817-594-0705, Fax: 817-594-1471.
(410 Lution Weatherford, TX 76087)

D. Other Supplements Often Used by Cancer Patients

1. Okra-Pepsin-E3, 1 after each meal for two months (depends on how much mucus is built up in your small intestine; see page 34, Cleansing the Small Intestine.)
2. Hydrochloric Acid (Mega Acid A or Beta-Z), 1 with each meal.

Minerals: Nature's Most Important Nutrients

Dr. Kelley, searching 50 years for the proper metabolic minerals, found them early in 2000, minerals small enough to go in and out of each cell. TheAngstrom Minerals included above are the blessing he has so long sought, one angstrom unit in size. Colleg Health Stores, LLC, 1-888-477-3618, 1-817-594-0705, Fax 1-817-594-1471, College (410 Lution Weatherford, TX 76087).

Protocol for Class I: Immune System Malignancies; Aids, HIV, etc.

Follow C above; *Metabolic Supplementation Support of One's Body Having Malignant Tumors.* You should substitute Formula A for Formula Ca+.

Protocol for Class II: Soft Tumors Malignancies; Hodgkin's, Leukemia, Lymphoma, etc.

Follow C above; *Metabolic Supplementation Support of One's Body Having Malignant Tumors.* You should substitute Formula L for Formula Ca+.

"Why on Earth Do I Have to Take So Many Pills?"

Metabolic Medicine's Cancer Cure Program® has succeeded with a high percentage of former cancer patients because it reverses the process of degeneration. You have cancer because you allowed your overall general health to degenerate; Metabolic Medicine's Cancer Cure Program® helps you to *re*generate. Dr. Kelley does not deny that his approach applies extreme measures. he maintains that extreme measures are required when you have allowed your health to fall so low that you have left yourself vulnerable to cancer. He has identified four major lines of defense against cancer: the pancreas; the immune system; mineral balance; calcium metabolism. All of them depend heavily on nutrition for their strength.

You take so many pills because Metabolic Medicine's Cancer Cure Program® leaves nothing to chance. You take so many pills in order to be sure that your glands will be totally supported, your immune system highly stimulated, and your body chemistry properly balanced. You take so many pill because the objective of Metabolic Medicine's Cancer Cure Program® is to turn your degeneration into your regeneration.

Additional Help Information for Cancer Victims

As brought forth throughout this book, you, the cancer victim, if you choose to be cancer free, you must take responsibility for the resolution of your own metabolic malfunctions. We can only provide you with information and bring to your attention what has been so successful in my own body and the bodies of thousands of others who have the courage, intelligence, wisdom and determination to address their own condition. HEALTH is a do it yourself lifetime procedure. However, you will need information, counseling, encouragement and know-how that others can provide for you from their own vast knowledge and experiences.

Helpful All Natural Remedial Procedures

Herbal Malignant Tumor Removal:

The herbal application of the Escharotic Salve can be the fastest, safest, and most thorough remedy available in removing a malignant tumor mass. The removal of the tumor mass may give you the valuable extra time needed for Dr. Kelley's Metabolic support. It is Dr. Kelley's opinion that the malfunction of the Pancreas causes a lack of enzymes in the system. As stated above, in a normal healthy person these enzymes digest the malignant tumor cells present in the body. A tumor mass drains the body of nutrients and releases toxins into the system. This protocol will help eliminate the tumor mass and the Metabolic Support protocol can help restore the body. If the tumor is not eliminated and the pancreas is not restored to health, the result could be fatal. For the bloodroot salve, call Dan Raber at 229-365-7141, or contact via email at danraber@sowega.net Review the website at www.skincanceranswer.com

Natural Vitamin Deficiency Replacement for Malignant Tumors:

Mr. G. Edward Griffin, outstanding investigative journalist, lecturer and author of many books, articles; producer of audio and video tapes on cancer and the political fraud and murder of the orthodox and alternative medical communities; gives us the most useful information available on natural vitamin deficiency replacement for use in treatment of malignancy. Mr. Griffin's book and video *World Without Cancer* are classics of health care information.

For a complete listing of available information needed by the cancer victim, contact Mr. Griffin's office, American Media, P.O. Box 4646, Westlake Village, CA 91359, telephone: 800-595-6596/805-496-1649, fax: 805-381-0191, www.realityzone.com

Chapter Four

Body Detoxification

In reality, a person rarely dies of cancer but always from starvation and toxicity. As the malignant tumor grows, it gives off waste products, which must be eliminated through the colon, liver, kidneys, lungs and skin. These waste products accumulate and gradually overburden the body. Most persons then die of toxemia.

Before any disease can be cured, the waste products and impurities must be cleansed from the body. The sooner this cleansing is done, the sooner the body can begin repairing itself. Dr. Kelley recommends that you begin the detoxification process even before you have the nutritional supplements in your possession. It is absolutely imperative that you carefully follow the detoxification process after the supplements begin stimulating the release of wastes and debris.

Scientists have calculated that persons have between 70 and 100 trillion cells in their bodies. This means we have over 70 trillion "garbage cans" needing to be emptied. In our culture we have neither made allowances for, nor taught ourselves, the proper techniques of emptying these waste receptacles. It is no wonder that the people of our nation are so sick! Proper and thorough detoxification is just as important as good nutrition for anyone who has lived in the mainstream of a modern technological civilization for 10 or more years, and especially for anyone who has developed symptoms of a chronic degenerative disease.

The intensive program of concentrated nutrients outlined in this book will begin to make nutritional factors available to the cells, which they may not have had for many years. Consequently, cellular metabolism will speed up and an increased amount of metabolic waste will be dumped into the bloodstream. Most people's organs of elimination do not function well enough to handle this increase in waste. If the waste accumulates in the bloodstream, one will not feel well and the cells will not be able to utilize the fresh nutrients being provided by the nutritional program.

When one eats food, it is digested in the mouth, stomach, and intestinal tract. In the intestinal tract, the digested food is absorbed into the bloodstream, which takes it close to each individual cell. The food, along with oxygen, is transferred into the cell, where nutrients are metabolized into energy, carbon dioxide, water, and waste products of metabolism. It is the accumulation of these wastes which frequently interferes with normal functions of the cells.

Principal factors necessary for a pure bloodstream are pure air, pure water, pure food, and the presence of oxygen brought in by exercise appropriate to your cardiovascular capacity.

As the cells produce metabolic debris, the blood carries it to the organs of detoxification. These organs are the liver, kidneys, lungs, skin, many of the mucous membranes, and the colon. If these organs of detoxification are themselves filled with debris, they, of course, cannot accept any more toxins. In such a case, the blood cannot accept further debris from the cells and, before long, there are 70 to 100 trillion garbage cans completely full. It is like the city dump being filled to capacity and not accepting any more garbage trucks. Then one's home becomes overloaded with garbage, which shortly interferes with normal functions of one's household. Before long, the entire community has become bogged down. "Clean blood," then, acting as a highway for the garbage trucks, is dependent upon the organs of detoxification.

Master Gland of Detoxification

The liver is the major organ of detoxification and also the most stressed by our modern lifestyle. One cannot live long without the heart, brain, kidneys, or pancreas, yet it is proper liver function which prevents these organs from becoming diseased. Here, in addition to metabolic wastes, is where environmental contamination, food additives, and all other chemical pollutants are removed from the body. You should be just as much or more concerned about the condition of your liver as about the condition of your heart. If you have had hepatitis, cirrhosis of the liver, infectious mononucleosis, or other liver damage, you should become very protective of this vital organ. The intake of anything that places undue stress on the liver should be eliminated entirely. Such a list would include: chemicals of any kind; drugs; synthetic foods; artificial food additives, such as flavorings, colorings, preservatives, emulsifiers, stabilizers, sweeteners; alcoholic beverages; carbonated beverages; hair sprays; chemical deodorants; and reheated vegetable oils used in frying, commercial pastries, and most fast foods. (Unrefined oils, or butter for sautéing, can be used without creating peroxides and free radicals, which are toxic to the liver.)

Major functions of this incredibly complex organ include:

- Metabolizing essential fats (cholesterol, triglycerides, lipoproteins) and thus preventing their accumulation in the bloodstream where they often form deposits on blood vessel walls (athero sclerosis).

- Synthesizing the bulk of necessary blood proteins.

- Breaking down and eliminating most drugs and environmental poisons.

- Secreting a fluid (bile) which stores in the gall bladder or the enlarged bile duct and empties into the small intestine.

The bile acts as a carrier for all liver wastes. It is also essential for the proper digestion and assimilation of fats and all fat-soluble nutrients such as vitamins A, D, E, K, lecithin, and essential fatty acids. The gall bladder is a hollow muscular organ which stores and concentrates bile and is attached to the undersurface of the liver. When a meal is eaten, especially if it contains some fats or oils, the gall bladder is stimulated to contract and should freely expel its contents into the small intestine to emulsify fatty nutrients for proper absorption and to allow poisonous wastes which the liver has removed from the body to be eliminated through the intestines.

Liver Congestion

Many people living in our society today, even those in their teens, fail to have free, unobstructed flow of bile from the liver and gall bladder in response to food entering the small intestine. Eating refined or processed foods, eating fresh food which is mineral- deficient because it is grown on depleted or chemically treated soil, lack of regular vigorous exercise, stress, multiple distractions during meals, and many other unnatural aspects of our lifestyle have combined to alter the chemistry of bile so that formation of solid particles from bile components is a commonplace occurrence among Americans. These solid particles remain in the gall bladder or the base of the liver for many years and become progressively harder, sometimes calcifying into "gallstones." Long before this occurs, however, metabolic problems are under way. When a significant number of solid bile particles accumulate, the free flow of the gallbladder is diminished, causing progressive stagnation and congestion of the liver. The body begins to suffer the effects of poor assimilation of fat-soluble nutrients, which may play a role in the development of eczema, psoriasis, dry skin, falling hair, tendonitis, night blindness, accumulation of calcium in tissues, and sometimes prostate enlargement in men. Hemorrhoids due to blockage of the portal vein draining the liver are often the result of this congestion.

Liver-Gallbladder Flush

The importance of cleansing the debris from the liver and gall bladder, thus keeping the bile free flowing, cannot be overemphasized. This cleaning can be effectively accomplished by doing the Liver-Gall Bladder Flush (a form of which at one time was widely used at the world-famous Lahey Clinic in Boston, MA), which is necessary even if one has had their gall bladder removed. The four basic active principles in this procedure are:

- Apple juice (high in malic acid) and ortho-phosphoric acid, which acts as a solvent in the bile to weaken adhesions between solid globules.
- Epsom salt (magnesium sulfate), taken by mouth and enema, which allows magnesium to be absorbed into the bloodstream, relaxing smooth muscles. Large solid particles which otherwise might create spasms are able to pass through a relaxed bile duct.
- Olive oil, unrefined, which stimulates the gall bladder and bile duct to contract powerfully, thus expelling solid particles kept in storage for years.
- Coffee enemas, which consist of a coffee solution retained in the colon, that activate the liver to secrete its waste into the bile, enhancing bile flow and further relaxing the bile duct muscle.

The Liver-Gall Bladder Flush is one of the most important procedures for persons over 15 years of age. For persons over 15 years of age and their physician gives approval, they should do this the first week of Metabolic Medicine's Cancer Cure Program, and should, with physician approval, repeat it every 2 months. The steps in doing this are not difficult and are as follows:

- For 5 days prior to the "Flush," consume as much apple juice or cider as the appetite permits in addition to regular meals. You may add a total of 90 drops of Phosfood liquid to the apple juice or cider each day. Nutritional supplements should also be taken during this time. The first preference for juice would be freshly juiced organic apples, and secondly, apple juice or cider (unsweetened and preferably organic if possible) purchased either at a health food or grocery store. A person should be sure to read the labels carefully and obtain a juice that has no additives whatsoever.
- If one is a severe hypoglycemic, is diabetic, or has difficulty tolerating the juice or cider, he or she may take 20 drops of Phosfood Liquid with each meal (60 drops daily) in water or some type of

juice other than apple. Due to the high acidity, it is wise that one brush his teeth or rinse out his mouth with Milk of Magnesia or baking soda solution after taking the ortho-phosphoric acid.

- At noon on the sixth day, one should eat a normal lunch.
- Two hours after lunch, 1 or 2 tablespoons of Epsom salt (magnesium sulfate) dissolved in 1 to 3 ounces of warm filtered, distilled, reverse osmosis or alkaline water should bc taken. The tast may be objectionalbe to some. If so, the mixture can be followed by a little citrus juice if desired (freshly squeezed if possible).
- Four hours after lunch, take a 1-quart coffee enema with one-fourth (1/4) cup of Epsom salt dissolved in it. This should be retained for 15 minutes and expelled. The coffee should be made as strong as one can tolerate but no stronger than 6 tablespoons of ground coffee per quart of water.
- Five hours after lunch, take 1 tablespoon of Epsom salt dissolved as noted in the dose 2 hours after lunch.
- Six or seven hours after lunch, fast if desired. However, it is preferable to have a fresh fruit salad with whipped cream, using as many fresh fruits or berries in season as possible. The whipped cream is necessary to cause gall bladder contractions. Use heavy, whipping cream as a dressing on the salad, whipped with a little raw (unheated) honey if desired. Eat as much as desired of the whipped-cream-covered salad. If fresh fruit is unavailable, frozen berries such as strawberries, blueberries, boysenberries, blackberries, raspberries, etc. can be used. These should also be covered with whipped cream and a large portion eaten. Take citrus fruit or juice after the cream and fruit meal, if desired. For hypoglycemics, the cream should balance the fruit. However, hypoglycemics should adjust the amount of salad eaten to their individual tolerance.
- (**Note:** Olive oil stimulates the gall bladder and bile duct to contract powerfully, thus expelling solid particles kept in storage for years. All juice should be freshly squeezed if possible):
- At bedtime, you have 1 of 3 choices.
    -Take one-half (1/2) cup of unrefined olive oil or 6 tablespoons of Formula F followed by a small amount of orange, grapefruit, or lemon juice, if the oil taste is objectionable.
    -Take one-half (1/2) cup of unrefined olive oil or 6 tablespoons of Formula F blended with one-half (1/2) cup of orange, grapefruit, or diluted lemon juice.
    -Take 4 tablespoons of unrefined olive oil or 4 tablespoons of Formula F, followed by 1 table spoon of citrus juice every 30 minutes until 6 ounces of oil have been consumed. This choice is preferable for those who are unusually weak or who have had gall bladder problems in the past. It has been found helpful to rinse the mouth with an alcohol base drink like sherry to cut out the residue of the oil taste. If an alcohol-base drink is unobtainable, try a natural carbonated drink or club soda. (**Do not swallow** the alcohol drink or the carbonated drink.)
- (**Note:** If you should vomit during the consumption of the oil and juice, the procedure should be continued until finished. It is not necessary to make up for the amount that was vomited. Nausea felt during this process usually indicates stimulation of the gall bladder and/or liver.)
- Immediately upon finishing the oil and juice (or while taking it), go to bed and lie on your right side with your right knee drawn up toward your chin for 30 minutes before going to sleep. This encourages the oil to drain from the stomach, helping contents of the gall bladder and/or liver to move into the small intestine.
- If you feel quite ill during the night, another strong coffee enema with one-fourth (1/4) cup of Epsom salt dissolved in it may be taken.
- If there is a strong feeling of nausea the following morning, you should try to remain in bed until

it subsides somewhat. Vomiting should not be forced.

- Upon arising, you must take another strong coffee enema with Epsom salt in it or 1 hour before breakfast, take 1 tablespoon of Epsom salt dissolved in 1 to 3 ounces of warm Wellness Water from the Alkalizer™ water instrument..

- If you continue to feel nauseous or sore in the upper abdomen even after the enema, a light diet of sprouts, fruit (raw or steamed), yogurt or kefir, and freshly extracted vegetable juices (especially with beet greens in them) should be resumed. If you find that the Metabolic Formulas cause discomfort immediately after the flush, they may be omitted for three days.

Helpful Hints

1. Taking one hydrochloric acid tablet at bedtime will help reduce any nausea during the night.
2. If you have a tendency to get nauseated from the oil, take 2 tablespoons of Aloe Vera juice after your doses of oil and citrus juice.
3. Placing a hot water bottle over the liver area (under the right ribcage) during the night also helps relieve nausea.

Note: One should not be frightened by the above references to nausea, vomiting, soreness of the abdomen, etc. Chances are that the symptoms will not be severe enough to cause vomiting or soreness of the abdomen, as this happens only very rarely. Many people complete this procedure with minimal discomfort, and nearly everyone feels much better after completing it. Flushing the liver and gallbladder in the manner described stimulates and cleans these organs as no other process does.

Oftentimes, persons suffering for years from gallstones, lack of appetite, biliousness, backaches, nausea, and a host of other complaints will find gallstone-type objects in the stool the day following the flush. These objects are light to dark green in color, irregular in shape, gelatinous in texture, and of sizes varying from "grape seed" size to "cherry" size. If there seems to be a large number of these objects in the stool, the flush should be repeated in 2 weeks.

Fasting

After the Liver-Gall Bladder Flush a fast may be started. The fast should last 1 or 2 days. The fast will give the body a rest and an opportunity to cleanse itself of much waste on the individual cell level. Each day of the fast one quart of fresh carrot juice and one pint of celery juice should be taken, along with all the Wellness Water desired. It is best to dilute the fresh juice with equal parts of Wellness Water.

It is important to remember that unless sufficient fluids are taken, the poisons become concentrated and are not eliminated in the natural way.

CLEANSING Small Intestine

If there were only one kind of pill that would help everybody, the cancer patient or otherwise, it would be "Okra-Pepsin-E3" made by Standard Process, Inc. This pill would probably do the nation's health more good than any other one pill, as it digests the mucus that coats the walls of many people's small intestine. Certain foods, such as pasteurized milk and many cooked foods, cause the mucus buildup on the wall of the small intestine (raw foods do not cause this mucus buildup). The mucus coats the villi on the wall of the small intestine. Villi are like tiny fingers that stick out from the intestinal wall to absorb nutrients from the digested food, which is primarily liquid. The mucus on the villi blocks the absorption of nutrients from the food. Sometimes the mucus becomes so thick and tough it is almost like a plastic film. Almost no nutrition can get through to the body. Persons with a severe mucus buildup could take $1,000.00 worth of supplements a month along with a good diet and still get almost no nutritional value from them. They would be starving and therefore would want to eat more food including protein which would lead to more of the pancreatic enzymes being used to digest the protein even though it could not be properly absorbed. When all the pancreatic enzymes are used up, there are none left in the blood to destroy cancer cells.

The okra is a sticky, gooey vegetable material that tends to stick the pepsin enzyme to the mucus on the intestinal wall long enough to digest some of the mucus. The E-3 is a powerful tissue repair factor and was originally developed for the patient with stomach ulcers or colitis.

If the Okra-Pepsin-E3 capsules are taken for 2 months, one after each meal (reducing the amount of capsules if diarrhea occurs), the mucus will gradually be digested. The blood can then receive more nutrients from the food, even if from a poor diet. Then, once a year, take the Okra-Pepsin-E3 capsules again for 2 months to keep the mucus from building back up. The mucus blockage varies with different people; sometimes it blocks minerals and larger molecules only, while in other people it partially blocks all nutrients.

While taking the Okra-Pepsin-E3 capsules, people who have heavily mucus-coated intestines might find mucus coming out with their stool, convoluted like the intestines. Dr. Kelley has had people who have been taking the capsules call him to say that they think they have just passed their intestines and what should they do. (He assures them it was not their intestines; it was ropes — or tubes — of mucus.)

One 37-year-old patient called Dr. Kelley to report that the Okra-Pepsin-E3 capsules worked a miracle by relieving reoccurring pain she had suffered with for years. (The pain would come and go apparently without cause and felt like bricks were pressing against her internal organs and lower back and at the same time her right side and leg would feel numb.) On the morning of the eighth day, after taking one Okra-Pepsin-E3 capsule with each meal for a week, she spent 45 minutes sweating, straining and pushing to have a bowel movement, and when it finally came out she could hardly believe what she saw — long, intertwined black ropes (or collapsed tubes) of mucus filled the toilet! She feels lighter now and has not had the pain since that day. (After this bowel movement and the disappearance of her pain she realized that there must have been a connection to eating a large meal and the pain — food passing through the intestine would push the mucus-coated intestine onto nerves, which caused the pain and numbness.)

The Okra-Pepsin-E3 is indicated for both underweight and overweight people. In both cases nutrients are not being absorbed. Even if they are taking enzymes to digest the food they eat, they absorb only the smaller carbohydrate molecules while the larger protein molecules are blocked. In underweight people the carbohydrates are used efficiently (burned for energy, not turned into fat), but the person becomes thin as they lose muscle mass from lack of protein absorption. In overweight people the carbohydrates are not used efficiently (they are turned into fat), and this causes them to become overweight as they also lose muscle mass.

Metamucil™ (Psyllium husks), one or two tablespoons daily, mixed with water or juice, may be taken to sweep the mucus out of the colon, once it is broken down by the pepsin in the Okra-Pepsin-E3 capsules. College Health Stores, LLC at 888-477-3618/817-594-0705, fax: 817-594-1471 (410 Lution Weatherford, TX 76087).

Cleansing The Colon

The Coffee Enema

A high, retention enema, using coffee, should be taken to aid in the elimination of toxic waste material from the body. The coffee enema should be taken daily for as long as one is on Metabolic Medicine's Cancer Cure Program®. After 37 years Dr. Kelley still takes his daily enema. The coffee enema is very stimulating to the liver and is the greatest aid in elimination of the liver's toxic wastes.

The coffee enema, besides stimulating liver detoxification, also has beneficial effects in cleaning the colon. Coffee is an excellent solvent for encrusted waste accumulated along the walls of the colon. The caffeine also directly stimulates the peristaltic muscle to contract more powerfully and loosen such deposits, which are occasionally visible as hard, black material and "ropes" of mucus. Gradually, as the protein metabolism of the body improves, the muscle tone of the bowel becomes normal and thorough evacuation is possible without the aid of the enema. Essentially, coffee enemas help the liver perform a task for which they were not designed — that of elimination in 1 or 2 years the accumulated wastes from many years of living in ignorance of the laws of nature.

At first, most people dislike enemas and have psychological barriers against them. Ignorance of the purpose and function of the enema, as well as misunderstanding of the proper procedure for taking it, bring about this aversion. I have observed, however, that the persons most opposed to enemas soon reverse their prejudices and become the most avid supporters of them! In many cases, the enema relieves distress and gives a sense of well-being and cleanliness never before experienced. The proper removal of toxins and debris from the colon is absolutely essential in all conditions of disease and ill health.

It is most desirable to take the coffee enema early in the morning and it may be repeated again in early afternoon and/or evening, depending upon the toxic condition of the body. Enemas using coffee in the afternoon or evening may interfere with sound sleep. If enemas are needed at these times, many patients prefer to use only warm pure water omitting the coffee. But it is better to take coffee at these times also, and a weaker solution to permit sleep would be better than not using coffee at all.

Organic Coffee for the Coffee Enema

Many people prefer to use organic coffee for their enemas. One researcher in Canada has produced and developed a special, effective blend of organic coffee beans from different parts of the world that produce a very effective coffee enema. This research has created the first cofee blended and roasted for enema use, s.a. Wilson's Therapy Blend Coffee. Scott Wilson, Blackstock Coffee Co.,

Inc., 14041 Old Scugog Rd., Blackstock, Ontario L0B 1B0, Canada, 1-905-986-1444, Fax 1-905-986-0738.

How to Make A Coffee Enema

- Just before bedtime each day, make a pot of coffee (1 quart). Unplug the coffeepot and allow to cool to room temperature.
- It is best to arise early enough each morning to allow time to take the enema in a relaxed, unhurried state.
- The coffee must be regular, non-instant, non-decaffeinated coffee. It must be prepared in enamelware, Corning Ware™, glass or stainless steel, or by the tricolator filter method. Aluminum or Teflon should not be used at any time! We have found the coffee unbilled or prepared via the "drip method" is preferable. Use 3 to 4 tablespoons of ground coffee to 1 quart of warm filtered, distilled, reverse osmosis or alkaline water should be used.

Avoidance of city water supplies (always chlorinated, which has been strongly linked to hardening of the arteries, and often fluoridated, which has been strongly linked to cancer and thyroid disease) is most essential to removing stress from the kidneys. Any water that enters the body should be from filtered, distilled, reverse osmosis or alkaline water should be used. This water should be used for cooking and drinking — and even for preparing enemas, since a significant portion of the enema water may be absorbed and filtered through the kidneys. Even if one has a well, it should not be assumed safe. Often toxic amounts of copper, cadmium, and lead are picked up from the plumbing, even if the well water is pure. It is best to purchase the Alkalizer™ water instrument. Remember, if one distills water from a city supply, one must remember that certain hydrocarbon contaminants have boiling point the same as that of water. The distiller should have a valve to permit their escape as they gasify. If not, they will concentrate in the distilled water and will need to be removed by filtering through activated charcoal.

One may purchase the Alkalizer™ water instrument from the College Health Stores, LLC at 888-477-3618/817-594-0705, fax: 817-594-1471 (410 Lution Weatherford, TX 76087).

If a coffee enema makes a person jittery, shaky, nervous, nauseated, or light-headed, the coffee solution is too strong. The amount of coffee can be adjusted from 1 teaspoon to 4 tablespoons per quart of water, as tolerance level permits.

- The high, retention coffee enema should consist of 1 quart of coffee, held for 15 minutes. Some people, children especially, can take and retain only a pint (2 cups) of enema solution at a time. If this is the case, one must take 2 enemas each time, one right after the other, and hold each for 15 minutes as directed.
- Upon rising each morning, plug in the coffeepot for a few seconds to bring the coffee to body temperature; unplug and take the morning coffee enema.

How to Take A Coffee Enema

A. Before the enema do some form of mild exercise if possible, such as walking briskly. If you are extremely debilitated and weak, this step will of course need to be omitted until strength returns.

B.   Attempt a normal bowel movement. The enema is much more effective if the colon has been evacuated. You should not become disturbed, however, if there are no regular bowel movements, or very few, during Metabolic Medicine's Cancer Cure Program®. In many cases, not enough bulk collects to instigate a normal bowel movement. When no normal bowel movements are forthcoming, the enema cleans the colon adequately.

•   Bulk formers such as Metamucil™ (or other brands of Psyllium Husks obtainable at drug or health food stores) taken as directed, or 2 tablespoons of miller's bran with each meal (obtainable at a health food store) are quite helpful in forming stools and thereby creating more normal bowel movements for those who take daily enemas.

•   After the normal bowel movement, if one is forthcoming, or before taking the coffee retention enema, most people find that taking an enema with 1 quart of warm Wellness Water is very helpful (do not retain this enema). This procedure begins the cleansing of the colon, removing large particles of residue and most of the gas. When it is completed, the coffee retention enema may be taken. The warm-water enema is optional and does not need to be taken if the coffee enema can be retained for the desired period.

•   Place 1 quart of coffee in your enema bag or bucket. You may use a Fleet enema bag, which is a disposable, large-volume plastic bag, an over-the-counter item from the local pharmacy or hospital supply outlet. This enema bag lasts about 2 years.

•   The enema tip on the end of the hose is not adequate to give a "high enema." Place a colon tube (DAVOL) size 24 French or 26 French or 28 French on the opposite end of the plastic tube from the enema bag. This colon tube is a soft, flexible, rubber-like tube around 30 inches in length. It follows the curves and flexure of the colon. The colon tube is usually inserted about 12 to 20 inches into the rectum. (Editor's Note: It is difficult today to find a colon tube. However, a plastic rectal catheter or tube about 18 inches long may be ordered from your pharmacy as an over-the-counter item.)

•   Allow the coffee to flow to the end of the colon tube, thus eliminating any air in the tube.

•   The colon tube should be lubricated with natural creamery butter, Vitamin E cream or other lubricant that does not contain additives or chemicals.

•   Insert the tube 12 to 20 inches into the rectum, if possible. This insertion should be done slowly, in a rotating motion that helps to keep the tube from "kinking up" inside the colon.

•   The enema bag should not be over 36 inches higher than the rectum. If placed too high, the coffee runs into the colon too fast and under too much pressure, causing discomfort.

•   Several positions can be used while inserting the colon tube. Squatting is one. There is also the knee-chest method, with chest and knees on the floor and buttocks in the highest position possible. Most people, however, find it easiest to lie on the left side until the solution is out of the bag or bucket. The enema should never be taken while sitting on the toilet or standing.

•   Some people's colons have kinks or turns in them that may prevent the tube from being inserted even 18 inches. Often, if a little bit of the solution is allowed to flow into the colon as the tube is being inserted, you may comfortably get past these kinks.

•   If a kink bends the tube too much and stops the flow of liquid, then the tube can be inserted only as far as it will go, still allowing the liquid to flow freely.

•   Sometimes, if you hit a kink that stops the flow of the liquid completely, the tube can be pulled out slowly just to the point where the solution is felt flowing again. Frequently, the tube can be pushed back in, past the turn that previously stopped the liquid.

C. Because of the shapes and formations of some people's colons or of course, if a child is being given the enema, it will be possible to insert the tube only a few inches; occasionally, this is a permanent situation. Often, however, as the colon is cleaned and healed, the tube can eventually be inserted further.

- The tube should *never* be forced when discomfort occurs.
- After the flow of the solution is completed, you may remove the colon tube, although it is not necessary to do so. Regardless of the position used up to this point, you should now lie on the left side for at least 5 minutes, then on the back for another 5 minutes, then on the right side for at least 5 minutes.
- Those who have excessive gas may leave the tube in the colon with the hose clamp open, allowing gas to escape through the enema container. Frequently, the coffee will go in and out of the enema bag or bucket until the gas is relieved.
- After the enema is retained for 15 minutes or longer, it may be expelled.
- You are now ready for the rest of your daily routine clean and refreshed!

Helpful Hints

- If you find you have a lot of gas and it is difficult to retain the enema, try putting 2 tablespoons of blackstrap molasses into your coffee solution.
- If you get a sudden gas bubble causing an urge to expel the solution, breathe fast through your nose using your abdominal muscles like a bellows; this usually helps the colon wall break up the gas bubble.
- If you find that a little coffee leaks out, place an old towel under your buttocks.

Intestinal Obstruction

Occasionally, the intestinal tract will become obstructed. Usually under these circumstances, no food or feces will come through. After a few days, people becomes extremely nauseated and start vomiting. They will be very sick and will normally run a high temperature. This should be watched quite carefully, for in such cases immediate emergency treatment is absolutely necessary.

You should never allow yourself to become extremely toxic. But, in order to distinguish between a healing toxic reaction and an intestinal obstruction, as soon as nausea or vomiting develops and no food is passing through, all supplements and food should be stopped for 5 days. Water and juice may be taken during this time. If there is no vomiting, food is passing through, and the temperature remains below 100 degrees, the diet and normal routine may be resumed, as you can assume there is no obstruction.

A point to remember is that you should not fail to cycle off the supplements routinely before reaching such a state of toxicity!

If, during the 5 days off the supplements with no solid food intake, you begin to vomit and have abdominal pain with a high temperature, your physician should be consulted to check for intestinal obstruction.

Kidneys

The kidneys, vital organs of detoxification, filter approximately 4,000 quarts of blood daily. The metabolic wastes, largely urea, are eliminated and the acid/alkaline balance maintained. Many drugs are eliminated through the kidneys, especially the common pain-killing drugs that can be extremely damaging to these organs. Such drugs include aspirin, phenacetin and acetominophen. People often do not experience any symptoms from loss of kidney function until 90% of the function is gone, and then the damage is irreversible.

The kidneys should be flushed each day with liberal quantities of fluid, wellness water, or fresh fruit and vegetable juices (preferably organic). Parsley tea is excellent for strengthening the kidneys. Those with kidney problems should avoid ordinary commercial teas and coffee as a beverage. Herbal teas are acceptable.

For those who tend to retain fluid, watermelon is an excellent diuretic. If the melon is organically grown, the rind should be juiced and sipped first thing in the morning and then the red fleshy part of the fruit may be eaten. Two mornings a week, one may take the juice of a whole lemon in warm wellness water as a diuretic (citrus should not be used more than 2 days a week, as it tends to upset the calcium-phosphorus metabolism if used more frequently). Shavegrass or horsetail tea is a good diuretic and also good for the skin and hair. An excellent diuretic salad may be made by combining cabbage and onions — finely sliced — with crushed raw garlic, parsley, and herbs like sage, cumin, and juniper berries, if available. Cover this mixture with very hot wellness water and place a lid over it for 10 minutes. Drain the mixture (the liquid is good to save for soup bases, grains, etc.) and squeeze a lemon over it. It can be eaten as is or refrigerated first and can also be mixed with other salads.

In extreme fluid retention, a physician may prescribe a diuretic drug, which is permissible, and the doctor will normally increase the intake of potassium to compensate for its loss due to the drug. In kidney disease the protein intake should be limited and extra vitamins and minerals taken.

Lungs

Life is dependent upon the adequate exchanges of gases in the lungs. The most significant are the removal of carbonic acid and the flow of oxygen into the blood. The lungs give off many other gaseous wastes. Sometimes before, but more frequently after the start of Metabolic Medicine's Cancer Cure Program®, patients or persons close to them may notice a foul odor on the breath. No amount of toothpaste or mouthwash will remove it for long, since it comes from the bloodstream. One can be assured, however, that this is only a phase and that the poisons are leaving the body.

Excessive accumulation of mucus in the nostrils and/or bronchial system, inhibits the detoxification functions of the lungs. Mucus-forming food should be avoided if mucus is a problem. These mucus-forming foods are principally dairy products, with the exception of butter and cream, and baked flour products. Anti-mucus foods such as raw onions and garlic, cayenne pepper, freshly ground black pepper, fresh ginger, and horseradish should be eaten liberally.

Skin

Most people overlook the skin as an organ of detoxification. But the skin is sometimes called "the third kidney," since many of its functions in fluid and electrolyte balance are similar to those of the kidneys. When great amounts of poisons flood the body, all systems are overloaded and this function of the skin is sorely needed. As the skin is utilized, all sorts of eruptions, odors, colors, and blemishes may appear. These conditions will disappear as the body becomes purified. You can quickly assess the relative efficiency of elimination through the skin by looking at your iris (the colored portion of the eye). The skin is represented by the outermost part of the iris. If the skin is very dark and dense, the condition is called a "scurf rim" in iridology, which means that the skin is relatively blocked as an organ of elimination. To open it up, skin brushing before a shower and vigorous use of a loofah sponge in the shower are recommended. A good quality vegetable-bristle, skin brush should be purchased from a health food store or pharmacy. Brush up the front of the body and down the back over all exposed skin surfaces, until a warm glow is felt. Take a warm shower and rub briskly with a loofah sponge (available in most health food stores) to remove the layers of dead skin loosened by the brushing. (We have found it best to take a hot shower each morning.)

Castile or other pure soap should be used — but in a minimal amount, since heavy soaping will wash off all the valuable skin oils and can cause the skin to overproduce oil in order to compensate. The hair should be shampooed frequently with a non-chemical soap or shampoo, which can be found in health food stores.

At the end of the shower turn the water to cool, then to warm. As you become accustomed to the temperature change, you may go from hot to cold and back several times. This exercises the tiny muscles in the skin, which control dilation and contraction of the pores. As they become stronger, they can respond better to the physiological demands of the body.

After the shower, sit in a tub of water with a cup of apple cider vinegar added, to restore and strengthen the acid mantle of the skin. Afterward, the body should be dried and rubbed briskly with a towel until a warm glow is felt.

Epsom salt baths may also be used to help draw toxins out of the skin. These baths are especially beneficial if one is going through a "healing crisis" and is especially toxic and feeling bad. Such a bath works best after the skin brushing and use of a loofah sponge. A tub is filled with warm to hot water and 4 or more cups of Epsom salt are dissolved in it. This bath is quite relaxing and good for tense, sore muscles, and may be taken as often as needed.

Every fourth night the cancer patient should be rubbed from head to toe with a mixture of olive oil and castor oil in equal parts. Then a hot soaking bath should be taken for 15 minutes to allow the oil to penetrate, followed by going to bed under heavy covers for about one hour to sweat the poisons out. Then a cleansing shower is taken. This procedure may be discontinued after three months.

Irrigating the Nostrils

Salt-water irrigation of the nostrils is helpful with nasal mucus and sinus congestion alike. If you cannot breathe through the nose, you are bypassing a crucial filtering mechanism which warms and humidifies the air, and which removes large amounts of smoke and dust before this air reaches the back of your throat. Mouth breathing places incalculable stress on the lungs, nearly equivalent to that of cigarette smoking if you live in urban pollution.

To irrigate the nostrils, dissolve 1 teaspoon of sea salt in 16 ounces of warm water in a bowl of appropriate size. While bending forward, block one nostril and place the other below the water surface in the bowl. The water should be gently pulled up the nostril until you can taste the salty mixture trickling to the back of the throat; then it should be blown out. This should be repeated with the other nostril and alternated several times.

Breathing Exercises

Breathing exercises should follow the cleansing of the nostrils. If done on a regular basis, these exercises yield tremendous benefits: Increase the body's supply of oxygen (which is the basic currency for repair and for burning up toxins); step up the removal of waste products and stagnant air from portions of the lungs otherwise unused; and exercise the diaphragm — which serves as a pump for the flow of oxygen and nerve energy.

Deep breathing yields a multitude of benefits through maximum use of lung capacity.

Rapid breathing is an energizing exercise, which promotes flow of energy into the lungs and digestive organs and should be done before meals, after being in a stuffy room, or whenever a lift is needed.

Alternate-nostril breathing has a calming effect on the nervous system and can be used effectively to overcome anxiety states and insomnia, and sometimes to relieve headaches.

Breath is the external manifestation of our life force. It *is* our very life. We can live for a while without food or drink, but not without breath.

Exercising

In almost every case of cancer, particularly those cases of long standing, the protein from the muscles has been used to maintain life. In other words, protein metabolism has been so poor that the body had to take protein from the muscles and, to a great degree, the muscles have been consumed.

After the cancer is destroyed, the muscles begin to rebuild. This rebuilding takes approximately three years. If the muscles are exercised strenuously during this time, a hernia may develop. For this reason we have found it best to replace strenuous exercise with a brisk walk at least once a day for three years following therapy.

DIAGRAM OF DIGESTIVE SYSTEM

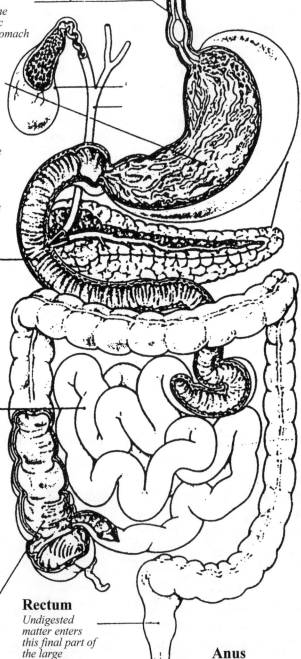

Esophagus

Food is carried down the esophagus by peristaltic action and enters the stomach

Stomach

The pancreatic enzyme must be in an enteric matrix. Food is broken down further by churning and by the action of hydrochloric acid and digestive enzymes secreted by the stomach lining. Food remains in the stomach until it is reduced to a semiliquid consistency (chyme), when it passes into the duodenum.

Duodenum

The pancreatin starts its functions. As food travels along the duodenum, it is broken down further by digestive enzymes from the liver, gallbladder, and pancreas. The duodenum leads directly into the small intestine.

Small Intestine

Additional enzymes secreted by glands in the lining of the small intestine complete the digestive process. Nutrients are absorbed through the intestinal lining into the network of blood vessels and lymph vessels supplying the intestine. Undigested matter passes into the large intestine (the colon).

Colon

Ox Bile is needed to help digest fats. Water in the undigested matter leaving the small intestine is absorbed through the lining of the colon. The residue passes into the rectum.

Pancreas

In some individuals, the pancreas does not produce enough of these enzymes all of the time, therefore supplementation may be a good idea as insurance to assure that there is no deficiency.

Rectum

Undigested matter enters this final part of the large intestine and is expelled.

Anus

Chapter Five

Metabolic Medicine's Cancer Cure Diet

About the year 424 B.C. Hippocrates, the father of modern medicine, made the statement, "Your food shall be your medicine and your medicine shall be your food." Try as we may, we have not been able to improve upon this basic truth, particularly when it comes to the successful treatment of the cancer patient. At least 86% of all cancer conditions could be adequately treated and/or prevented by diet alone.

It never ceases to amaze me at the number of learned, as well as ignorant, persons who scoff when diet is mentioned. They all seem to believe that no matter what is placed into the body, by some magical process, it makes for perfect health. Yet these same people are quite fastidious and concerned about what, how and how much food is fed to their pedigreed dogs and cats and their registered cattle and horses. It is ironic that they cannot see that their own health is equally dependent upon a proper balanced nutritional process.

Kelley Almond Diet

From the first printing of this book in 1967 we have called our diet the "Kelley Almond Diet" because the principal protein is almond and vegetable protein.

Raw almonds are a good source of protein and may be used as directed: several almonds at breakfast and several almonds at lunch.

A mixture of raw almonds, cashews, pecans, filberts, Brazil nuts, walnuts, sunflower seeds, pumpkin seeds, and sesame seeds is recommended to supplement protein during the first six months, when meat proteins are severely restricted. This mixture should be eaten any time up to 1:00 p.m.

Cashew nuts are desirable, especially if the patient is also suffering from hypoglycemia (low blood sugar).

Nuts, seeds, and grains should be stored in closed containers in a cool location. Refrigeration is best if space allows.

Some enzyme researchers do not recommend the use of raw seeds or nuts, claiming that the enzyme inhibitors in the seeds or nuts make proper digestion difficult. This is true in one sense — if raw nuts and seeds were swallowed whole without masticating them, a person could not digest them properly. But if nuts and seeds are chewed well or soaked overnight (in Wellness Water) the activity of enzyme inhibitors is greatly reduced or nullified.

Should you have difficulty chewing whole raw almonds, you may substitute two tablespoons of pure raw almond or sesame seed butter.

Phase One: Protein

We have maintained throughout this treatise that cancer is nothing more than a pancreatic enzyme deficiency. The greatest cause of this deficiency is the amount of cooked protein (mutated amino acids) fed into the body. The pancreas simply cannot manufacture enough enzymes to digest the large volumes of pasteurized milk and cheese and cooked meat we eat and have any enzymes left over to digest the foreign protein we know as cancer. If people would not eat protein (animal) after 1:00 p.m. (or eat the animal proteins within a 4-6 hour period), 86% of cancer in the United States could be eliminated.

However, cancer patients should never give up all protein, as they might be tempted to do when first learning that too much protein in the diet prevents the pancreas from ridding the body of cancer. The pancreatic enzymes themselves consist of protein (amino acids), and unless the body is fed adequate protein, the pancreatic enzyme production will stop and the cancer tissue will make a rapid growth. The total withdrawal from protein has been the fallacy of many cancer diets, such as the "Grape Cure." This is also the reason these diets have worked so well for the first few months — no protein — thus freeing the pancreatic enzymes to digest the cancer. Yet, over prolonged periods of total abstinence from protein, the pancreas fails. Proper balance and regulated intake are the answers.

Timing

It is not only imperative that the correct kind and quantity of protein be eaten, but of equal importance, it must be taken at a specific time. We have found that regular proteins should be taken at breakfast and lunch only. When this time frame is strictly observed, the pancreatic enzymes, used in digestion of protein, are used only about 6 hours, leaving 18 hours for production of pancreatic enzymes to digest cancer tissue.

If the average cancer patient is carefully observed, it will be noted that they start the day with protein—a glass of milk, ham and/or bacon and eggs, or milk with cereal. By mid-morning they are ravenous and have a candy bar, peanuts, doughnuts or sweet rolls with a soft drink or coffee. For lunch they normally have a roast beef sandwich or chicken fried in "trans-fatty acid" vegetable oil, or a hamburger. By mid-afternoon they are again hungry and have been attacked by low blood sugar, so perk themselves up with coffee or a soft drink. Dinner consists of a charbroiled steak or a piece of roast beef or other cooked meat with white flour gravy and cooked-to-death vegetables. For dessert there is ice cream or pie á la mode with another glass of milk. It is impossible for the pancreas to produce enough enzymes under these conditions.

Eggs

Eggs are an unusually good source of protein — well-balanced and the standard by which all protein is evaluated. Eggs have all the essential amino acids in proper proportions. The cancer patient may have two eggs (preferably raw) each day at anytime.

Proper preparation of eggs is of vital importance. The eggs must be heated in the shell. We bring our eggs to a temperature of 140° F. to 160° F., (the normal temperature of hot tap water), for five minutes before cracking them. This cooking method destroys an enzyme just inside the membrane under the shell that prevents the biotin in the egg from functioning normally. When biotin functions properly, it greatly reduces the cholesterol risks of eating eggs.

After preheating before cracking them, the eggs may then be eaten, as you prefer them. Raw and soft-boiled eggs are the most preferable, though it is not absolutely necessary to eat them in these forms. In keeping with the use of as much raw food as possible, a good procedure is to eat the eggs raw in a blended drink of some kind, flavored to taste.

A group of research doctors and dentists who, for at least a dozen years, had eaten two eggs daily (properly prepared as above), as part of a well-balanced nutritional program. Tests conducted on these people showed no increase in cholesterol. In fact, there was a significant decrease in the blood serum cholesterol level of each individual.

Misconceived beliefs of the orthodox medical world about eating cholesterol-containing foods have caused countless people to be unduly alarmed about cholesterol levels and the associated possibility of heart attacks. These misconceptions, carried on from the early 1950's, have been proven false.

Liver

Liver, a wonderful energy food, cannot be surpassed as a blood builder and is especially crucial for leukemia and lymphoma patients, as their blood is unusually weak. However, all cancer patients can benefit from the intake of raw liver before noon each day. In the mid 1960s, when Dr. Kelley was told he was in the final stages of pancreatic and liver cancer, he found that raw liver blended into carrot juice gave him strength when everything else he ate made him feel ill.

Raw organic, antibiotic-free and hormone-free liver contains a multitude of live enzymes, amino acids and other intrinsic factors that science has not yet identified, which are destroyed when the liver is cooked. (References to "intrinsic" or "unidentified" food factors are fairly common in nutritional literature. They result from clinical reactions, which cannot be linked to known nutrients. Raw liver for cancer patients is an excellent example of powerful therapeutic, but unexplained, effects.) No supplements or drugs can take the place of raw liver; none are in any way comparable in their effects. Eating raw liver ensures thorough digestion and the replacement of expended nutrients, promoting excellent health.

Raw liver is best if it is organic, antibiotic-free, hormone-free and not irradiated. However, if this type of raw liver is unavailable, 3 to 6 TBS of fresh muscle meat, steaks and ground, may be eaten, raw also, are acceptable, even if you buy them at regular markets. Organically grown and not irradiated is always more nutritious and preferable. But if organic is not available, commercial is healthier than none. At least 3 and no more than 6 heaping tablespoons of raw liver should be taken daily.

Chewing the liver is best for proper digestion. However, if masticating it is too objectionable, it will digest well even swallowed whole, if sliced into small enough cubes and if adequate hydrochloric acid and enzymes are taken.

Two methods people find suitable for preparing liver:

- The liver can be sliced about ¼ inch thick, placed on a cookie sheet, and frozen. After freezing, it can be cut into ¼ inch cubes. Use plastic sandwich bags, putting 3 to 6 tablespoons of frozen cubed liver in each bag and storing them in the freezer for daily eating. This frozen liver may be chewed or swallowed whole, followed by a sip of juice if desired. Some prefer to allow the liver to thaw and then to place a spoonful at a time in the mouth and chew it or swallow it whole with a sip of juice.

 • Liver may be placed in a blender with carrot, pineapple, or tomato juice (and seasoning of preference if desired), blended, strained to remove the fiber if preferred, and used as a morning "pep-up" drink.

Meat (Cooked and Commercially Produced)

The cancer patient will want to give up cooked and commercially produced meat such as beef, pork, lamb and fowl immediately (except for raw liver — see above). Cooked meat is harmful for the cancer patient, as the very same enzymes used in its digestion are needed for fighting and digesting the cancer. All natural, self-made enzymes your body can produce should be used to fight the cancer. Commercial meat should be avoided for another reason; it has a high female sex hormone content. For commercial reasons most animals, especially beef and fowl produced in the United States have been fed large quantities of hormones. Since an overabundance of female sex hormones initiate cancer, meat of this type should be excluded from the cancer patient's diet.

After being on Metabolic Medicine's Cancer Cure Diet for 9 to 12 months, when the tumors are under control, you may gradually resume consumption of meat as long as your metabolic type requires it (see Chapter VIII, Metabolic Typing — Discovering Your Personal Nutritional Needs) and adequate enzymes and hydrochloric acid are taken to digest it.

If and when you do go back to eating meat, it will be extremely wise to make every effort to find a source that can provide meat, which has been produced without chemical feed, hormones, antibiotics, and pesticide residues.

Protein After 6 Months on Cancer Diet

After the first six months on Metabolic Medicine's Cancer Cure Diet® the cancer patient must increase the quantity of protein in his diet. At this time not less than 60 grams of protein daily should be included in the diet. You should, of course, continue all the above approved protein, but now you may include (or increase) such proteins as those found in deep-sea fish, all forms of seeds, nuts (except peanuts), nut butters, whole grains, whole-grain breads, and home-made, raw (unpasturized) goats' milk yogurt and/or buttermilk.

Seeds and Sprouts

Raw seeds and sprouts are good foods for cancer patients and may be eaten after 1:00 p.m. We freely use brown sesame, sunflower and pumpkinseeds. Many people enjoy sprouted seeds, such as alfalfa and mung beans, buckwheat, wheat and soybeans.

The most "living foods" are sprouted seeds. When seeds are soaked in water, their protective enzyme inhibitors are removed and the enzymes, which have been "asleep," become active, and in three days the nutritional values of the seeds are increased tremendously. The seeds also become much easier to digest.

For the best in nutrition, be sure to eat your sprouts raw and eat as many as you desire.

Beans

Dry beans of all types are a good source of food for the cancer patient and may be used 2 or 3 times a week at anytime of the day. The best way we have found to prepare beans is to cook them at a temperature of 200° F. Place 2 cups of dried beans (washed) in a bean pot to which is added 5 cups of water, 5 garlic cloves, 2 tablespoons of olive oil, 1 teaspoon of sea salt or kelp, and 1/8 teaspoon of cayenne pepper. Place the pot (covered) in an oven overnight at 200° F.

Phase Two: Vegetable and Fruit Juices

Vegetable Juices (Fresh and Raw)

The second most important phase of our cancer diet is that of fresh raw juices. At least one quart of carrot and one pint of celery juice should be taken each day. As much other fresh raw vegetable juice in volume may be taken as desired. One should consider alfalfa, beet, cabbage, cucumber, dandelion, endive, lettuce, parsley, potato, spinach, and turnip juice. Vegetable juices are the builders of the body. Juice is better than the whole vegetable because so much energy is used to digest the whole vegetable. Juice has a proper balance of vitamins and minerals in a concentrated solution. We recommend that the juice be made fresh and used immediately.

Fruit and Fruit Juices (Fresh and Raw)

Fresh raw fruit and fruit juices are the cleansers of the body. The cancer patient may eat as much as desired of fresh raw fruit or fresh fruit juices. Small amounts of dried unsulfered fruit may also be taken.

Fresh Fruit and Raw Vegetable Salads

The cancer patient may eat, in addition to his fresh raw vegetable and fruit juices, all the fresh fruit and fresh raw salad he or she can hold. These are good for lunch or dinner meals. The body needs bulk, as it is necessary to keep the digestive tract in good working order. For at least the first eight months on Metabolic Medicine's Cancer Cure Diet®, lemon should be used in preference to vinegar on salads. Unrefined, organic flaxseed oil may be used as salad dressing. Dr. N. W. Walker's books, *Fresh Vegetable and Fruit Juices* and *Diet and Salad Suggestions,* are recommended reading for every cancer patient.

Phase Three: Whole-grain Cereal

We have found that it is desirable in building the body to eat a mixture of raw whole grain cereals for breakfast each morning.

Mix together well in a large container one pound of each of the grains and nuts below. Store in refrigerator (if too large a quantity is mixed for your refrigerator, it will keep in a cool, dark pantry).

Multi-Grain Porridge

Objective: to obtain as many different nutrients as possible from as many different seed and grain gene pools as possible from as many different sources (fields) as possible.

Contents by equal weight of **Organic:**

AMARANTH	PUMPKIN SEEDS
BARLEY	RICE, BROWN LONG GRAIN
BARLEY FLAKES	RICE, BROWN SHORT GRAIN
BUCKWHEAT GROATS	RYE BERRIES
CORN MEAL BLUE	SPELT BERRIES
CORN MEAL YELLOW	SUNFLOWER SEEDS
KAMUT	TRITICALE FLAKES
MILLET	WHEAT, HARD RED SPRING
OAT GROATS	WHEAT, SOFT PASTRY

Adding almonds, English walnuts and bananas makes a complete tasty meal.

Directions

Daily at bedtime:
- Grind 1/3 cup porridge grains in seed mill.
- Add 1 cup boiling water; stir well.
- Let soak at room temperature overnight.
- For breakfast add fruit, concentrated fruit juice and/or unheated honey to taste.

Hot Porridge

After two years this porridge may be cooked in a double boiler as in oatmeal or other grains—best in a double boiler or on low heat.

Phase Four: Flax Seed Oil

Take 2 tablespoons per day of unrefined, fresh flaxseed oil for the first month of Metabolic Medicine's Cancer Cure Program® and 1 tablespoon per day from the second month of the program to completion. (Formula F provides Essential Fatty Acids—Essential Fatty Acids must be provided in the diet, as the human body cannot make them.)

Johanna Budwig, a German researcher, did the lion's share of the early work on flax oil and its therapeutic uses in the early 1950s. Blood samples from healthy and sick people were systematically analyzed, and the findings tabulated. According to her, blood samples from people with cancer, diabetes, and some kinds of liver disease consistently lacked Essential Fatty Acids (EFAs). She claims that blood from people with other diseases did not show this severe deficiency and that healthy people's blood always contained EFAs. If cancer is a deficiency disease brought on by lack of EFAs, she reasoned, a diet high in EFAs should alleviate at least some of the cancer patients' problems.

Unrefined flaxseed oil, in practice, inhibits tumor growth and is useful in the natural treatment of cancer. EFAs from refined oil, on the other hand, help promote tumor growth (due to trans-fats present in *all* American commercial vegetable oil). *All* oils except unrefined, fresh olive and flaxseed oil are forbidden on Metabolic Medicine's Cancer Cure Diet.

Note: Fat that has not been heated above 96° F. in the form of unsalted raw butter, raw eggs, raw cream, the fat in and on raw meats, no-salt-added raw cheeses, avocados, fresh coconut and stone-pressed olive oil is acceptable on Metabolic Medicine's Cancer Cure Diet®. These fats are the easiest to digest, assimilate, and utilize and aid the body in binding with toxins and carrying them to the bowels and out of the body.

The Golden Rule

The Golden Rule of Metabolic Medicine's Cancer Cure Diet® is: "Take nothing into the body that has been cooked or processed except items mentioned." Eat no **processed** food for the first 6 months of Metabolic Medicine's Cancer Cure Program.

The juicer is the most important appliance in the kitchen of a cancer patient. If necessary, sell the stove and buy a good juicer.

The enzymes in cooked foods have been destroyed or changed into a different compound (amino acid). Cooked food can only be used as food and not as enzymes, for it has no life. For example, if you plant a raw potato it will grow. If you boil a potato and plant it, it will not grow, but will rot. Many enzymes are destroyed at 107° F. and almost all are destroyed at 140° F.

When people eat anything processed they are not only eating "dead food" (those in which the enzymes have been destroyed), but are adding a second destructive force to his body, the destructive force of food preservatives. This may not be too significant for a normal healthy person, but for the cancer patient, it may mean life or death. The liver must detoxify, destroy, or metabolize all foreign substances from the body. When one eats foods with preservatives, it adds an extra burden upon the liver, which the cancer patient cannot accept.

Milk

The cancer patient must give up pasteurized cows' milk forever, except in the form of raw (unpasteurized), homemade yogurt, and for a while must avoid raw milk too, except raw (unpasteurized) goats' milk. Cows' milk, like meat, has too high a protein content and pasteurization compounds the problem as it alters or mutates the protein. Pasteurized cows' milk requires too many pancreatic enzymes for digestion.

Also, an animal cannot produce milk unless the female sex hormones are present in extra- large quantities; this causes too many hormones in milk for the person who has cancer.

But if raw goats' milk is available, it is advisable to take 4 to 8 ounces of raw (unpasteurized) homemade goats' milk (goats' milk is similar to humans' milk) yogurt each morning for breakfast. This will supply the intestines with adequate helpful bacteria and is acceptable because the yogurt bacteria predigest the milk protein when added to it.

After following this diet for 9 to 12 months and if raw goats' or cows' milk is available, 9 to 12 ounces per day may be taken at any time during the day.

Peanuts

The cancer patient will also want to give up peanuts. First, the peanut is not a nut, but a legume. Second, the peanut also has too much protein for the cancer patient. Third, it has been found that a fungus grows on peanuts, which produces aflatoxin. To stimulate cancers in experimental animals cancer researchers use aflatoxin.

Processed Foods

White Flour

All concentrated foods are extremely hard on the liver and should be given up. White flour and all products containing white flour should be avoided; these are not only concentrated carbohydrates, but almost always have preservatives added.

Use fresh whole-wheat bread, made from wheat grown free of all pesticides (another liver- destroying chemical). The essential vitamins are oxidized within 3 days at room temperature; hence, the need for grinding only as used. Freshly ground flour or freshly made whole-wheat bread may be safely stored deep in a deep freeze for about a week. It is best, however, to use it within 3 days.

White Sugar

The cancer patient will also want to give up all white sugar and white sugar products. The concentrated carbohydrates are hard on the liver, but more important in relation to cancer, are hard on the pancreas. The pancreas, as noted earlier, is the first organ to be protected at all costs. White sugar has been processed (refined) and all the vital minerals are taken out. Cancer patients are always deficient in minerals.

For those who have a sweet tooth, these organic foods may be eaten as desired: Dates, date sugar, figs and raisins obtained from a health food store. These foods are free of toxic pesticides and are not harmful to the pancreas or liver. A cancer patient may also eat pure maple syrup or unheated honey, in that order. The first is preferable because it has a higher mineral content.

Soy Products

Soy products, except lecithin, should be used sparingly for two reasons: First, the protein content is too high for the cancer patient; second, soy products tend to upset the delicate acid/alkaline balance of the body. Eating soy products may be resumed when Dr. Kelley's Pancreas Self-Examination Procedure is negative (see page 17).

Other Improper Foods

Lemon juice should replace vinegar altogether. Vinegar is too harsh on the delicate mucus membrane of the alimentary canal. Also, the ingestion of large quantities of vinegar causes the digestive tract to become too acid and thus, decreases the efficiency of the pancreatic enzymes and the digestive processes. For at least the first 8 months on Metabolic Medicine's Cancer Cure Program®, lemon juice should be used in preference to vinegar on salads. Unrefined, organic flaxseed oil may be used as salad dressing.

For the period of intensive detoxification and treatment, tea, coffee, soft drinks, chocolate, liquor, tobacco, pork, and white rice should be avoided. These also place additional stress upon the liver and pancreas, as they are being detoxified.

Chapter Six

Structural and Neurological Stimulation

While the body is being properly detoxified and nourished, the nerve supply to the pancreas and liver should be considered.

A specific organ works only when told to by a nerve, chemical, or pressure stimulation. Upon taking careful histories, we found a number of cancer patients who had had blows to the head or spine. We feel that such experiences change the nerve impulses to the various organs. If pressure on a nerve to the pancreas causes it to cease sending impulses to the pancreas, the pancreas will turn off and wait until the nerve tells it to work again. If the nerve is destroyed, or for some reason never sends a message, the pancreatic function will be greatly impaired.

Probably the best way to reactivate the nerve enervation is through some form of manipulative therapy such as osteopathic manipulation, chiropractic adjustments, or physiotherapy. We have found it advisable to have such a weekly manipulative treatment, for at least the first nine months of cancer treatment. The regular body massage that people are familiar with are not as good but also helpful.

Neurological stimulation can sometimes be increased or simulated by hormone therapy, but this technique must be performed under the direction of a very highly skilled clinician. If the services of such a physician are unavailable in your area, the human growth hormone Eden Gh-1 (over the counter hormone prepartion) is very helpful and available from College Health Stores, LLC at 888-477-3618/ 817-594-0705, fax: 817-594-1471 (410 Lution Weatherford, TX 76087).

Temporomandibular Joint (TMJ) Equilibration

Temporomandibular Joint (TMJ) is such a mouthful that dentists like to use just the initials. It is the name of the joint just in front of the ear where the lower jaw hinges, one on the right side and one on the left. One or both of them are being forced out of place, may lead to being such distressing or painful conditions as earache, headache, head noises, clicking sounds, dizziness, nervousness and even mental troubles.

For such ailments, doctors may prescribe hot and cold packs, diathermy, massage vibration, rest, surgery, psychological treatment or drugs. While all of these remedies are useful at times, they often do not bring permanent relief *if stress in the joint is the real cause of the trouble.*

When the cause *is* stress in this joint in front of the ear, as it often is, a safe and highly successful dental treatment may be the solution. This treatment is known as "equilibration" (pronounced ee-quil-i-*bray*-shun); it simply means equalizing the muscle forces to restore the lower jaw and its joints to their normal unstrained or neutral positions.

How do the joints get out of adjustment in the first place? It might be from a blow on the chin, a muscle spasm, or opening the jaw too wide (as when biting or yawning). But the most common cause is chewing with teeth that come together in a wrong way.

Dentists refer to this condition as "malocclusion."

We close our jaws in chewing food, of course — and most persons also press their teeth together one or two thousand times a day between meals in swallowing. If the teeth do not meet properly, the pressures on them during chewing and swallowing may force the lower jaw into a strained position that pinches the joints in front of the ears.

If you could see through the skin and get a side view of the TMJ, you would see how the mandible, or lower jaw, hinges to the skull. The joint consists of a ball-and-socket arrangement, with the ball being a rounded mass of bone in the back part of the lower jaw that fits into a socket at the base of the skull. When you open and close your jaw, this "ball" rotates in its socket, and — if the teeth push the jaw too far in any direction — the soft tissues between the bones are pinched.

One trouble that sometimes follows this pinching is a slow loss of hearing, says one authority on TMJ disorders. He cites the case of a man who was losing his hearing and had been wearing a hearing aid for two years before he learned of equilibration. He had neither noticed any discomfort at the joints in front of his ears, nor that his teeth were not meeting properly, but suspected that his teeth might somehow be causing stress. His dentist made the necessary changes on the chewing surfaces of his teeth. Three days later the patient's hearing had improved to such an extent that he discarded his hearing aid and he has not needed it since. That was nine years ago, and his hearing is still good.

Not all patients respond so quickly or so completely, of course, and there are many other causes of deafness, the authority points out — but pressure at the TMJ should not be overlooked.

Besides hearing trouble this authority says that stress in the TMJ can cause neuralgia, stiff neck, running and itching ears. He tells of a woman who suffered from itching ears so much that in company, she often had to excuse herself from the room to scratch her ears. X-ray pictures showed both temporomandibular joints to be out of normal adjustment. After her dentist corrected the chewing surfaces of her teeth, the itching gradually left. (X-ray pictures showed that the joints are now in proper adjustment.)

It is not uncommon for stress in the TMJ to bring on head noises. A patient who wore artificial dentures in which the teeth were out of adjustment, forcing the left side of his jaw backward until the joint on that side was under considerable stress, experienced almost immediate relief from roaring sounds in his ears after being treated by his dentist. This was several years ago, and the roaring sound has not returned.

Although the connection between stress in the TMJ and the troubles cited is not fully understood, it is known that there is a connection, because when the condition in the joint is corrected, the troubles often disappear.

How does the dentist restore the joints to a normal condition of equilibrium? As part of the treatment he may change the slopes of the natural or artificial teeth or make the teeth higher or lower to bring the chewing muscles into proper working relationship. Sometimes he reduces pressure on the front teeth, so that the chewing forces fall more on the back teeth. (If the ball parts of the lower jaw have been pushed too far up into their sockets, this "pivoting" allows them to settle down again into their normal relaxed positions.)

As the TMJ authority notes, one advantage of equilibration treatment is that it can be done in the dental office and, in many instances, saves the patient from the more radical treatments of surgery or the injection of chemicals into the joints. Quite often, in fact, equilibration is the only treatment needed.

As with other treatment, *preventing trouble* is an important aim of TMJ diagnosis. Because TMJ stress sometimes builds up gradually, with the patient suffering no inconvenience at first, the lower jaw and its joints are often checked for equilibrium to *prevent* trouble.

Dentists, Physicians Team Up to Treat TMJ Disorders

Dentists and physicians all over the world are teaming up for diagnosis and treatment of TMJ disorders. (One physician-dentist reported improvement in over 85% of more than 1,000 patients treated with pivoting; another physician-dentist team reported that 52 of 54 patients obtained relief from dizziness after equilibration.)

In 1955 many dentists and physicians from the U.S. and abroad organized as the American Equilibration Society to further more intensive study of the TMJ and related structures.

CranioSacral Therapy

This therapy is a gentle, non-invasive, hands-on approach that focuses on the craniosacral system of the body. This system consists of the membranes and cerebrospinal fluid that surround and protect the brain and spinal cord. It extends from the bones of the skull, face and mouth — which make up the cranium—down to the sacrum, or tailbone.

This system has been effective in evaluating and treating problems associated with pain and dysfunction, lowered vitality, and recurring infections. The light touch employed in this approach encourages your own natural mechanisms to improve the functioning of the brain and spinal cord, to dissipate the negative effects of stress and to enhance general health and resistance to disease.

Craniosacral therapy by osteopaths, chiropractors and dentists has proven to help people who complain of ringing in the ears (tinnitus) and some forms of hearing loss.

Chapter Seven

Spiritual Attitude

If your cancer has caused you to stop, think, pray, and know God better, it has been a blessing to you.

If your cancer has caused you to realize the importance and magnificence of this temple wherein your soul dwells, you have been doubly blessed.

If your cancer has caused you to look within and ask Christ to dwell within you, you have been thrice blessed.

Often physical infirmities come to us for such a purpose; this was true in my own case. The still, small voice within spoke out to guide and teach this Child of God.

Not all who have cancer will overcome the condition. Many will not believe that such a simple treatment will work. Many will not have the opportunity to hear about and try the procedure. Many will come too late with a temple (body) too weak to respond. But, I pray with all of you my friends, that you will learn a beautiful lesson and learn it well. I did.

Each of God's children is in an experience in their school (earth) each doing their very best. Jesus said, "Judge not, that ye be not judged." (7 Matthew 1); "This is my commandment, That ye love one another, as I have loved you." (15 John 12).

If your cancer has taught you spiritual truth, you have gained much. I pray with and for you that at this point, you have come to the realization that your spiritual decision to get well or not to get well is your own responsibility. If you decide to go home early, rejoice, for the Father prepares a place for you. Those of you who have loved ones who have made this decision, rejoice with them and send them on their way into God's care.

If you decide to stay in school a little longer, this is also good and it should now be easier. If you are to operate as a perfect being in perfect health, then you must have a perfect attitude. You must become aware of the spiritual power within that is greater than you, the still, small voice within.

If you are of the many millions of people who have been told that you have cancer and that your days are numbered, then it is you who must be interested enough to seek out the truth of your condition. You have read many things in this treatise, which bring new thinking to a very old disease.

Since we are dealing with the metabolic approach to cancer, we must consider not only the physical, but also the mental and spiritual laws of God. We need help from those around us as well as the God power within to reverse our thinking, and attain that balance which creates a healthy physical being.

As stated in previous chapters, half measures will avail you nothing. You are at the point where you must ask God for guidance. Following are the suggested steps, as a method of spiritual recovery:

- Accept the fact that you are afflicted with a symptom (malignant cancer) and that recovery is possible.
- Establish a faith in a power greater than yourself and know that with His help you can regain health and harmony.
- Make the decision to turn your will and your life over to the care of God.
- Conduct a complete self-analysis to better understand your own emotions.

- Admit to God, to yourself, and to others the exact nature of what you find to be your shortcomings.
- Be willing to give up what you are doing wrong.
- Seek through prayer to improve your conscious contact with God. Pray only for knowledge of His will for you and the strength to carry that out.

Having had a spiritual awakening as a result of this action, practice these principles in your every thought.

Just as the body must be purged and cleansed, so must the emotions and spirit be purified. This is a comparatively simple task to accomplish, but do not lull yourself into believing that it is an easy task. Rigorous self-discipline and the ability to grasp and develop a manner of living with complete honesty in all of your actions and thought are necessary. You must become strong-willed to be a winner in accomplishing that which you set out to do for yourself. You will look for all the good in everything and refuse to accept any negation.

STOP! LISTEN!

Listen with your heart
He's been knocking softly
Just ask Him to come in

He made you
He loves you
He's always been there

He's the truth
He not only has
The answers, He's the
Answer for you

The Lord's the Light
Through Him you'll
see the Father

He's knocking
He's knocking
Just let Him come in
and His gift to you
Will be Heaven

Mrs. John Mark (Dei) Kelley

Chapter Eight

Metabolic Typing

What, you may ask, is metabolic typing? Metabolic typing is discovering your personal nutritional needs

Without knowing your metabolic type, you are guessing as to what foods and supplements you should take. This chapter explains how you can develop a personalized nutritional program that gives you the results you want.

You may be following a program of the best foods, the best supplements, and plenty of exercise — but how do you *know* that those really are the *best* foods for you? Each of us is different and has a different metabolism.

Many of the world's leading scientists including, for instance, biochemist Dr. Roger Williams, author of many excellent and well-known books such as *You Are Extraordinary*, and Nobel Prize Winning Physicist, Dr. Linus Pauling, have proven this through their own research.

Basic Metabolic Considerations

Individuals are classified into 10 basic types, named "Metabolic Types One through Ten." By classifying each person into their own proper type, it is possible to determine accurately what vitamins, minerals, foods, and other supplements would best support their own body chemistry. Equally important, it is possible to know what supplements and foods they should **not** have. With the knowledge of these factors, it is possible to design a program that has the fullest potential. All people fall into one of the metabolic types, that is to say, they fall into one of the basic ways the body functions. Each person's body takes in food, water and air. How a person uses these raw materials to maintain life differs from one person to another. This function of maintaining life is called metabolism and is normally defined as the sum total of all the chemical reactions occurring in the body.

The Nervous System

The body has two nervous systems— the voluntary nervous system and the autonomic nervous system.

Voluntary

The voluntary nervous system is that part of the brain and nerves that are under the control of the conscious mind. Activities that you have definite control over, like making decisions, walking, speaking and the like are controlled by the voluntary nervous system.

Autonomic

The autonomic nervous system is that part of the brain and nervous system that carries on the functions of the body that we have very little or no conscious control over. The autonomic nervous system controls such activities as our heartbeat, respiration and reflexes (like what happens when a person sits on a tack).

The autonomic nervous system regulates the basic life-sustaining functions of the body such as the turning on and off of glands and organs, maintaining the acid/alkaline balance of the blood, saliva, and urine, digestion of food, balancing glandular functions, turning the cells on and off, and stimulating and retarding the body and its parts.

The autonomic nervous system is the master regulator of metabolism. It determines how efficiently and effectively the body uses food, water and air.

The autonomic nervous system consists of two divisions, one division the sympathetic nervous system and the other division, the parasympathetic nervous system. Each of these two divisions sends messages in the form of electric current to the different parts of the body. There is a nerve from each of the divisions to each part of the body.

Sympathetic Nervous System

The sympathetic nervous system sends messages that in general accelerate or speed up our activities.

Parasympathetic Nervous System

The parasympathetic nervous system sends messages that in general retard or slow down our activities.

Three Groups—Ten Types

The autonomic nervous system plays a major role in the classification of the metabolic types. The 10 metabolic types have been arranged into 3 groups:

1. **Group A**, which includes the **Sympathetic** Dominant Metabolic Types: One, Four, and Six.

2. **Group B**, which includes the **Parasympathetic** Dominant Metabolic Types: Two, Five, and Seven.

3. **Group C**, which includes the **Balanced** Sympathetic/Parasympathetic Metabolic Types: Three, Eight, Nine and Ten.

Group A: Sympathetic—Vegetarian Types

Group A metabolizers are classed as Types One, Four and Six. These types have very strong or dominant sympathetic nervous systems. These types have very strong functions of the brain, pineal, anterior pituitary, parathyroid, thyroid, and adrenal medulla glands; heart, bone, muscle and connective tissue, kidneys, gonads (ovaries or testes), and uterus or prostate. Their muscles are usually quite well developed and show good muscle tone. Their hearts normally beat a little fast. Constipation is an ever-present plague. Frequently insomnia is a problem. Tension, hyperactivity and drive are their plight.

Sympathetic Metabolizers Are More Prone To:

Achlorhydria

Acidosis

Acne

Alcoholism (to slow down)

Anemia

Angina pectoris

Anxiety

Appetite, diminished

Arteriosclerosis (hardening of arteries)

Arthritis, rheumatoid

Bleeding (slow to stop)

Blood pressure, high

Boils

Bones, pain in

Bowel movement every 2-3 days

Breathing, rapid & irregular

Buerger's Disease

Bursitis

Cancer

Canker sores

Carbohydrate metabolism, slow

Caries (cavities)

Cataracts

Chorea

Circulation, poor from muscle tension

Colitis, ulcerative

Conjunctivitis

Constipation

Cystitis

Dehydration

Diabetes

Digestion, slow

Dizziness

Earache

Emotional instability, easily upset

Endurance, lack of

Energy reserve, low

Epilepsy

Extremities, cold from tension

Eyes, dry

Fat metabolism, slow

Febrile diseases

Food, feels like rock in stomach

Function well in hot climate

Gag easily

Gas, sweet odor

Glossitis

Goiter

Gout

Halitosis

Heart attacks, several

Heartburn

Heart rhythm, regular & fast

Headaches; migraine, tension

Healing; bones, fast

Healing; tissues, slow

Hemorrhoids

High temperatures

Hyperirritability

Hypertension

Hypochlorhydria

Indigestion

Infections, bacterial

Insomnia

Ketosis
Kidney, infections
Kidney stones
Legs, restless at night
Mastitis
Moods, frequent severe changes
Mouth, dry
Myocarditis
Nephritis
Nervous strain
Numbness
Oxygen metabolism, poor
Pain, unusual sensitivity
Pellagra
Peyronie's Disease
Photophobia
Pneumonia
Protein metabolism, poor
Pulse, fast

Purpura
Rheumatic fever
Sensitivity to light
Sensitivity to shots, vaccinations
Skin, dry, thick
Sour stomach
Stools; dry, light in color, ribbon-like
Sweating, little
Teeth, pearly white
Tinnitus aurium
Tonsillitis
Tremors, muscle
Ulcers, gastric
Uremia
Urinate, infrequently
Veins, varicose
Vincent's infection
Vision, hard to focus

Typical Characteristics of Sympathetic Metabolizers

A lot of "get-up-and-go" or drive
Actions usually explosive
Anger easily
Bowel movements normally light in color
Cannot recall dreams
Crave sweets, fruits
Difficulty in falling asleep
Diminished or lacking appetite
Dislike of fatty or oily foods
Dry mouth
Ears pale and light
Eating at bedtime interferes with sleep
Enhanced ability to concentrate
Enjoy exercise—"exercise nuts"
Enjoy vegetables
Extremely active
Eyelids opened wide
Eyes tend to protrude from sockets
Faces usually pale
Fingernails have severe cross ridges
Firm muscle tone

Food feels like a rock in the stomach
Gag easily
Gums are pale or light
Hair is dry
Impatient, irritable
Irregular breathing
Jumpy and Nervous
Lack of endurance
Like to make decisions
Low energy reserve
Pupils of eyes are usually large
Rapid breathing
Seldom depressed
Seldom dream
Sensitive to light
Severe indigestion
Skin easily forms "gooseflesh"
Skin is dry
Skin unusually soft and velvety
Soles of feet are soft and uncallused
Strong emotions

Strong feeling of sexual passion   **Thin flat chests**
Suffer from cold, usually   **Underweight, usually**
Thick and ropey saliva   **Violent reaction to unexpected noise**
Thick eyebrows   **Weak dreams, if dream at all**

Nutritional Guidelines for Sympathetic Dominant Types

Of this group, metabolic Type Six's require the most nutritional support, the greatest number and strength of vitamins, minerals, enzymes and other nutritional factors that help the vegetarian type. Type One metabolizes require the second greatest nutritional support and also need the support that slows down the sympathetic nervous system and speeds up the parasympathetic nervous system. Type Four metabolizers need the least nutritional support of this vegetarian class — they are the closest of the three to becoming balanced type metabolizers.

For nutritional support, Sympathetic Dominant Metabolizers most often need: Vitamin D; Vitamin K; Ascorbic Acid; Biotin; Folic Acid; Vitamins B1, B2 and B6; PABA; Niacin; Potassium; Magnesium; Manganese; Zinc; Chromium; Hydrochloric Acid; Pancreatic Enzymes and Amino Acids. Each of the vegetarian Types (One, Four and Six) need these supplements, but each type needs different amounts and different ratios.

Metabolic Type One

Type One metabolizers come the closest of all the types to being purely sympathetic dominant people. One of the chief characteristics of Type One metabolizers is that they can burn carbohydrates slowly. Their bodies utilize the carbohydrates poorly and they are able to maintain their blood sugar level with very little fluctuation. If anything, their blood sugar level stays a little elevated. With this condition, they can eat mostly fruits and vegetables, maintaining their health and feeling well. These people are what are commonly called vegetarians. They very seldom if ever crave meats (except fish) and when they eat meat, they usually feel groggy and have a loss of energy. These people do not do well on lamb, venison, beef, sardines or salmon. They can do quite well on up to 100% of their diet raw. They should stress the following foods: whole grains including spaghetti, macaroni, breads, cereals; raw (unpasteurized) goats' milk, eggs; white fish. They may use spices, 2-3 cups of coffee (non-instant), herbal tea, or an occasional alcoholic beverage or sweet dessert (made with unrefined sugar or raw, unheated honey). They enjoy and do well on nuts and seeds; rice; fruits and vegetables like apples, apricots, bananas, berries, grapes, oranges, pears, plums, grapefruit, asparagus, lima beans, beet tops, cucumbers, sprouts, lettuce, collards, dandelion greens, kale, mustard, turnip greens, spinach, and any leafy green vegetable.

Metabolic Type Four

Type Four metabolizers are people who have strong sympathetic nervous systems but not nearly as strong as the Type One's. Type Four's are a little more balanced or non-strict vegetarians. These people usually have a genetic background of their ancestors coming from around the Mediterranean Sea — Spanish, Italian, Greek, Israeli, Arabic, etc. Type Four's burn or metabolize their carbohydrates and sugars somewhat faster than the Type One's. The Type Four's that tend toward having diabetes can normally control it with diet alone.

To maintain optimum health, Type Four's do well on fish, chicken, turkey, other fowl, beef (two times a week), almost all vegetables, a little fruit, sprouts, some citrus, eggs, and raw, (unpasteurized) goats' milk. Most American "vegetarians" fall into this class. Type Four's generally need about 60% of their food raw. They normally do not need as much nutritional support in the form of nutritional supplements as the Types One and Six.

Metabolic Type Six

Type Six metabolizers are people who are basically sympathetic dominant. They fall into the vegetarian class of metabolizers. Type Six's are poor metabolizers — that is, they take in their food and nothing much happens. Their bodies do not utilize their food, they get very little energy from it and are generally sickly. Their assimilation or utilization of food is about 20% of normal. They almost always feel bad or not up to par. Type Six's need about 60% of their food cooked. They need a great deal of supplemental nutritional support and require more hydrochloric acid, vitamins, minerals, enzymes, etc. than either Types Four or One.

Type Six metabolizers should give care to the intake of whole and complete natural foods. All refined, processed, synthetic foods and additives must be avoided at all times. Type Six people do best when they stress the following foods in their diets: adequate amounts of fruits and vegetables including lettuce, green vegetables, onions, radishes, potatoes; whole grains including spaghetti, macaroni, breads; gelatin and other desserts made with raw sugar or unheated honey; natural jams, jellies, ice creams, mushrooms, nuts, seeds, and seafood and fowl, which should be preferred over other meats.

Group B: Parasympathetic—Carnivore Types

Group B metabolizers are classed as Types Two, Five and Seven. These types have very strong or dominant parasympathetic nervous systems. These parasympathetic metabolizers have strong function of the posterior pituitary, hypothalamus, parotid, sublingual (saliva) and adrenal cortex glands; stomach, spleen, duodenum, pancreas, liver, small intestine, colon, lymph and immune systems. Their digestion is very good. They are not constipated, but to the contrary, tend toward loose stools and diarrhea. They have poor muscle tone. They are in general lethargic, slow, and fall asleep easily. They usually have a good reserve of strength.

Parasympathetic Metabolizers Are More Prone To:

Acids, cravings for	**Atherosclerosis**
Alcoholism (to raise blood sugar)	**Bladder, loss of control**
Alkalosis	**Blackouts**
Allergies	**Bloating**
Appetite, excessive	**Blood pressure, low**

Arthritis; hypertrophic, osteo
Asthenia
Asthma
Cold sores
Colds; flu, gripe
Colitis, mucus
Coughs, chronic
Cough up mucus
Cramps
Dandruff
Dermatitis
Diarrhea
Digestion, fast and strong
Diverticulitis
Drooling
Dropsy
Drowsiness
Eczema
Edema
Emphysema
Energy, gain after eating meat
Energy, loss after eating sweets
Fat metabolism, good
Fatigue, chronic
Fever blisters
Gas, foul
Gingivitis
Growling gut
Gums, bleeding
Gums, receding
Hair, oily
Hay fever
Headaches; eyestrain, hypoglycemia
Healing; bones, slow
Healing; tissues, fast
Heart attack, massive
Hepatitis
Hernia
Herpes simplex
Herpes zoster (shingles)
Hiccoughs

Bowel movements, easy to start
Bone breaks
Brucellosis
Histamine reactions
Hives
Hoarseness
Hydration
Hypoglycemia
Infections, viral
Intermittent claudication
Jittery feelings
Leg ulcers
Leukemia
Leukopenia
Lymphoma
Melanoma
Nausea, from eyestrain
Obesity
Osteoporosis
Oxygen metabolism, good
Periodontoclasia
Phlebitis
Poison ivy or oak, strong reaction
Postnasal drip
Protein metabolism, good
Psoriasis
Pyorrhea
Sex problems, impotence
Skin, itching of
Sleepwalking
Sluggishness
Sneezing attacks
Stomach pain, excessive hydrochloric acid
Telangiectasia
Tingling in extremities (from deposits in vessels)
Ulcers, duodenal
Urinary incontinence
Urination, sudden urges
Vision, easy to focus
Warts

Typical Characteristics of Parasympathetic Metabolizers

Actions are relaxed, calm, firm and positive
Appetites, above-normal
Cough frequently
Crave butter
Crave fatty meats
Crave salty food
Deep cough often
Desire fatty foods like cream sauces
Desire to be cautious
Difficulty in holding urine
Digestion, good
Dislike exercise very much
Dream frequently
Dreams are vivid and often in color
Ears, pink or flushed
Eating at bedtime makes them
feel better
Eating fruit makes them feel jittery
or jumpy
Emotionally stable
Energy elevated after eating meat
Energy loss after eating sweets
Excess saliva
Extremely sluggish
Eyebrows thin and scanty
Eyelids droopy or saggy
Eyes sunken

Bowel movements, easy to start
Chests, Enlarged, Round
Eyestrain, causing headaches
Faces, flush easily
Fall asleep quickly
Feel better and satisfied when eating meat
Gums, dark pink or bluish
Hard to get going in the morning
Intestines rumble and growl a lot
Little fear
Little "get up and go"
Marked endurance
More than one bowel movement per day
Mucus, frequently cough up
Often feel sad or dejected
Oily skin
Prefer large egg and bacon breakfasts
Recall most dreams
Ruddy complexions — good face color
Seldom get angry
Slow breathing rates
Slow to make decisions
Strong hunger pains
Urinate several times a day

Nutritional Guidlines for Parasympatheic Dominant Types

Metabolic Types Two, Five and Seven need some of the same nutritional support as do the vegetarian types, but for the most part, need entirely different vitamins, minerals and foods.

Type Seven metabolizers need more nutritional support than types Two and Five. Type Two metabolizers have such strong parasympathetic dominance that they need almost as much support as Type Seven's. Type Five metabolizers are more balanced, and their supplemental support is not as much as that of the Types Two and Seven.

Parasympathetic dominant metabolizers most often need such nutritional support as: Vitamins E and B-12; Niacinamide, Pantothenic Acid, Choline, Inositol, Calcium, Phosphorus, Calcium Ascorbate, Bioflavonoid Complex, Zinc and Ribonucleic Acid. These metabolizers should eat at bedtime enough to carry them through the night. They should not eat leafy green vegetables or take large quantities of the B vitamins.

Metabolic Type Two

Type Two metabolizers come the closest of all the types to being purely parasympathetic-dominant people. One of the chief characteristics of Type Two metabolizers is that they burn carbohydrates very rapidly. Their pancreases work so well that carbohydrates and sugars burn or metabolize so rapidly that these people have a tendency to develop hypoglycemia — low blood sugar. When they eat only fruits, vegetables and sweets, their blood sugar rises and drops many times a day and their energy goes up and down like a yo-yo. When Type Two's eat carbohydrates and sugars, which are metabolized quickly, they become weak and shaky after a spurt of energy.

Type Two metabolizers must have meat — preferably fatty, heavy, high-purine meats such as lamb, beef, salmon, and sardines. They are usually the people who order their steaks very rare. By eating these fatty meats, they slow down their carbohydrate/sugar metabolisms and feel they have eaten something that will "stick to their ribs." Their energy is released at a normal rate and they do not suffer the ups and downs energy-wise that fruits and sweets cause them to have. Normally, these metabolizers do not care much for sweets. They do well on root vegetables, cabbage, Brussels sprouts, cauliflower, carrot juice, and beans. They enjoy butter, cream, Danish pastries, cream puffs and foods with cream or butter added. They can do well by adding a small amount of whole grains.

Type Two people do poorly on leafy green vegetables, candies, fruits, sweets, high carbohydrate diets and sugar pastries. They should limit the B vitamins and intake of potassium supplements. Type Two metabolizers usually have a genetic background from German, Scandinavian and Northern European ancestry.

Metabolic Type Five

Type Five metabolizers are those persons who have strong parasympathetic nervous systems, but not nearly as strong as those of Type Two metabolizers. Type Five metabolizers are more toward the normal or balanced metabolism. They can tolerate a wide variety of foods. Type Five metabolizers do well on beef or lamb several times a week, seafood, salmon, tuna, raw (unpasteurized) goat cheese, avocado, beans, peas, lentils, celery, carrots, asparagus, butter, whole grain cereals and breads, some nuts and occasionally Danish pastry and raw (unpasteurized) goats' milk cheesecake.

Type Five metabolizers are not as prone to hypoglycemia as are the Type Two metabolizers. However, Type Five's can easily develop hypoglycemia if they indulge in too many candies and sweets. Many Americans fall into this class and do not do well as vegetarians.

Metabolic Type Seven

Type Seven metabolizers are the sickly, weak, inefficient parasympathetic metabolizers. Their bodies do not utilize their food well and as a result, they function poorly. They almost always feel bad or sickly, functioning sluggishly. It is difficult for them to maintain adequate nutrition in their individual body cells. Their body chemistry systems are quite inefficient and more than normal supplementation must be maintained at all times. Care must be given to the intake of whole and complete natural foods. All refined, processed, synthetic food and food additives must be constantly avoided.

Type Seven metabolizers are encouraged to stress the following foods in their diets: seafoods, sardines, salmon, brains, liver, heart, meat gravies and soups, non-colored unprocessed (unpasteurized) goat milk cheeses, beans, lentils, carrots, celery, butter, and cauliflower. Small amounts of Danish pastries, raw (unpasteurized) goats' milk cheesecake and an occasional alcoholic beverage may be taken. Type Seven metabolizers function best on purine meats such as salmon, tuna, beef, lamb, and wild game. These meats should be preferred over others and used whenever possible and practical. Care should be given to adequately detoxify the bodies of these metabolizers.

Group C: Balanced Sympathetic/Parasympathetic Types

Group C metabolizers are classified as Types Three, Eight, Nine and Ten. These types have balanced autonomic nervous systems. The sympathetic and parasympathetic nervous systems work well together in a normal balance of glandular activity and metabolic function. Group C metabolizers have balanced metabolisms, which are neither strongly meat-eating nor strongly vegetarian — they fall in the middle. They are both vegetarian and meat eating. Metabolizers in this category have the greatest freedom in what they can eat. Indeed, they enjoy and thrive equally on foods from both the vegetarian and meat-eating categories.

The balanced metabolizers burn their food neither too fast nor too slow. This is one of the reasons they do equally well on all varieties of food.

Balanced metabolizers generally need such nutritional support as Vitamins A, B-1, B-2, B-6, B-12, Niacinamide, Vitamin C, Bioflavonoids, Vitamin E, Folic Acid, Biotin, Pantothenic Acid, PABA, Calcium, Phosphorus, Magnesium, Manganese, Chromium and Zinc. Each of the balanced Types Three, Five, Nine and Ten needs these supplements but each type needs different amounts and in different ratios. They also require extra amounts of hydrochloric acid and pancreatic enzymes.

The balanced metabolizers can suffer from the conditions and disorders of either the vegetarian groups or the carnivore groups of metabolizers. They are prone to the following conditions and have the following characteristics, all of course, in moderation and generally not to the extreme.

Balanced Metabolizers Are More prine To:

Catch cold occasionally	**Occasional acne**
Coated tongues sometimes	**Occasional asthma attacks**
Digestion, fairly good	**Occasional cold sores**
Hay fever once in a while	**Occasional emotional upsets**
Infection once in a while	**Occasional fever blisters**
Maintain normal weight	**Occasional headaches from eyestrain**
Normal appetite	**Occasional hiccoughs**
Normal blood pressure	**Occasional indigestion**
Normal blood sugar— not diabetic or hypoglycemic	**Occasional itching skin**
Normal cholesterol level	**Occasional nausea**
Normal pulse rate—72-80 per minute	**Occasional rash or hives but not often**

Normal reactions to insect stings or bites
Normal skin texture—not too rough
and not too soft
Rumbling or growling of intestines sometimes
Seldom get motion sickness
Seldom have diarrhea

Occasional stomach ache
Occasional sweating

Seldom have insomnia
Seldom have spells of sneezing
Sour stomach sometimes

Typical Characteristics of Balanced Metabolizers

Actions are occasionally extreme or explosive
Normal alertness
Occasionally get angry
Occasional periods of fatigue
Sometimes experience belching
Normal bowel movements
Eyes are set normally in sockets
Normal thickening on soles of feet
Average size chests
Face colors are normal—not white or red
Sometimes have stomach pains
Seldom have constipation
Like a wide variety of food
Sometimes have dreams
Have a fair amount of drive
Hair is not too oily or too dry
Skin is not too oily or too dry
Like fruit, but also like meat
Normal endurance
Eyelids — eye slits normal
Fall asleep within a reasonable length of time
Normal amount of sexual passion
Don't mind exercise when there is time to do it
Gums have normal color tone —not too
light or too pink
Seldom have hoarseness
Don't get hungry between meals
Stable but occasionally run out of energy

Have coffee occasionally
Normal initiative and energy
Normal stools — not hard or loose
Very seldom need laxatives
Get started in morning without too
much trouble
Occasionally cough up mucus
Once in a while do things on impulse
Sometimes have a sense of ill health
Eyes have very little sensitivity to
strong light
Like all kinds of salad dressings
Saliva is normal—not too thick or thin
Occasionally need extra sleep
Occasional splitting of nails
Seldom, if ever, have mood changes
Handle stress fairly well
Voice is normal — not low or high
pitched
Don't worry much
Normal size bowel movements
Skin is not too thick or thin
Occasionally have reaction to shots or
injections
Handle quite a bit of pain
Fair muscle tone
Don't get excited easily

Balanced Metabolizers

Balanced metabolizers have different needs and requirements depending upon which type. Generally, however, they do well on a large variety of food.

Metabolic Type Three

Type Three metabolizers are balanced metabolizers; that is, their sympathetic and parasympathetic nervous systems are functioning in balance equally well. However, Type Three metabolizers come with bodies that are very inefficient. No matter what foods or supplements they take in, they are generally only going to use about 10% to 15%. Type Three metabolizers find it difficult for their individual cells to obtain adequate nutrition. All refined, processed, synthetic foods and food additives must be avoided at all times. Type Three metabolizers of necessity must take larger quantities of nutritional supplementation to maintain their nutritional health than any other type. They must eat food prepared in such a manner as to be easily digested. They should have a wide variety of foods, which enables them to get the wide spectrum of nutrients their bodies require.

Type Three (and Six and Seven) metabolizers are generally those with the poorest health. They have to keep constant vigilance over their diet and supplements. Generally they have inherited weak, defective bodies and very rarely will they ever have good health and feel really well if they are not extremely cautious.

Unfortunately, due to the stress of modern living and agribusiness, more and more Americans who have inherited good bodies have so exhausted and destroyed their bodies that they are now functioning in the Type Three (or Six and Seven) range. It would take supreme effort to rebuild and repair these bodies and put them back into normal optimum health again.

Metabolic Type Eight

Type Eight metabolizers account for the greatest number of people. More Americans are Type Eight than any other metabolic type. Type Eight metabolizers have fairly healthy bodies. Their bodies can adapt to a wide variety of stresses, yet remain stable. Their autonomic nervous systems also have a wide range of adaptability. Type Eight people need a wide variety of foods each day which permits them to attempt to obtain a large variety of nutrients required to operate their bodies efficiently. Nutritional supplements, like their food, must cover a wide spectrum.

Metabolic Type Nine

Type Nine metabolizers are in the balanced class — their sympathetic and parasympathetic nervous systems work equally well. This type is the most difficult to understand. If these people had a choice, they would always prefer cooked food. Working with these people through the years has led to the conclusion that they truly cannot do well on raw foods. Evidently, they have mutated to the point that they need cooked food to be satisfied. They generally require 70% cooked food and can comfortably handle 30% raw food. Type Nine metabolizers do best when they can eat at a Smorgasbord three or four times a week. In other words, if they eat a little of everything, they function best.

Metabolic Type Ten

Type Ten metabolizers are the people with balanced and super-efficient metabolisms. They need a wide variety of foods and supplements, but do not require a large quantity of anything. Their bodies are so incredibly efficient that they need only small amounts of food. If they eat a normal meal, they feel more than satisfied. They can eat half as much as any other metabolic type. They do well on any food but often prefer raw fruits, vegetables, whole grains and unpasteurized goat cheese.

Recap of Ten Types of Metabolism

Vegetarian

Type 1 — **Needs no animal products at all. Can live entirely on fruits, vegetables and nuts.**

Type 4 — **Needs some animal products such as fish, chicken, eggs and unpasteurized goat cheese several times a week.**

Type 6 — **Combination of Types 1 and 4, but has horrible metabolism. Needs more food to make up for lack of absorption.**

Carnivore

Type 2 — **Needs meat up to 14 ounces a day, preferably beef. Has little or no energy unless they eat meat.**

Type 5 — **Needs meat to feel good, but less often, perhaps 2-3 times a week.**

Type 7 — **A cross between Types 2 and 5 but with a horrible metabolism.**

Balanced

Type 3 — **Has horrible metabolism. Only absorbs 15% of what is eaten. These types often feel so bad they often wish they were dead.**

Type 8 — **Normal balanced metabolism. Can eat and benefit from all foods, provided they are wholesome.**

Type 9 — **Needs 70% cooked food in diet. Hates raw food.**

Type 10 — **Super-efficient metabolizer. Needs very little food and sleep, yet feels terrific.**

Dr. Kelley's Self-Test for the Different Metabolic Types®

Dr. Kelley developed his Self-Test for the Different Metabolic Types to help bridge the gap of research to practical application. He realized that the overall state of health of this nation could no longer be maintained acceptable unless the nutritional needs of the people were brought into immediate and sharp focus. No one (doctor or patient) knows what a well-balanced meal is. Doctors have neither been trained along these disciplines, nor have the time or inclination to educate themselves in these areas.

In order to make the most efficient use of research data, they must be related and applied directly to each individual to meet his specific needs. The problem then arises as to which data are significant for each patient. Dr. Kelley had to develop a system to accomplish this. It was decided that the most practical system would be an extensive questionnaire: Dr. Kelley's Self-Test for the Different Metabolic Types®. The test is bound in a book that contains hundreds of health questions, including complete instructions so you can score the results yourself (the results are compiled on an as-you-go basis during the completion of the questionnaire).

Taking the time (it takes a few hours) to complete the questionnaire will tell you: Whether you are a meat-eater, a vegetarian or have a balanced metabolism; which types of meats, fruits, and vegetables you should eat; and what supplements you should take, and, perhaps even more important, which you should avoid.

When you complete the questionnaire and follow the directions at the end of the book for scoring your answers, you will know where your body, at the present time, is functioning. There are three main metabolic types (Vegetarian, Carnivore and Balanced), and a number of sub-types (three in Vegetarian, three in Carnivore and four in Balanced). Each person will know exactly which of the three main types they are functioning in and also which sub-type.

After you follow the nutritional guidelines at the back of the questionnaire for your metabolic type for a few weeks or months, you will want to take the Self-Test again to determine if your metabolism has switched to another type. You should recheck your metabolic type every six months to a year, because it can change. If and when it does, your diet and supplemental program will have to be changed accordingly.

As you improve your blood chemistry, it is possible for your nervous system to go into balance—giving you a balanced metabolism. This can take years, or it may never happen.

However, I would not worry if it does not happen. As long as you are healthy and functioning normally—that is what counts.

Order Dr. Kelley's Self-Test for the Different Metabolic Types at College Health Stores, LLC at 888-477-3618/817-594-0705, fax: 817-594-1471 (410 Lution Weatherford, TX 76087).

Metabolic Type Spiral

Metabolic Efficiency

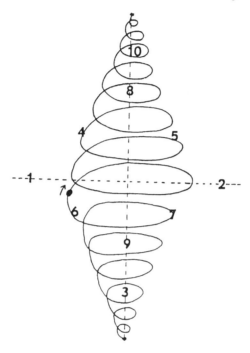

Metabolic Inefficiency

Shown above is the Metabolic Type Chart. This chart shows all 10 metabolic types and their relationship to each other, their sympathetic or their parasympathetic dominance and their metabolic efficiency.

On the left side are listed the sympathetic dominant types 1, 4, and 6. On the right side are listed the parasympathetic types 2, 5, and 7. And in the center column are listed the balanced types 10, 8, 9 and 3; these have a little of both sympathetic and parasympathetic dominating.

These 10 types are arranged on the Metabolic Type Chart on what might be called two sliding scales — one of them running horizontal and the other running vertical.

The horizontal scale runs from the extremely sympathetic type 1 to the more balanced but still sympathetic type 4 to the balanced type 8 to the parasympathetic type 5 to the extremely parasympathetic type 2. Ideally, one should have a more balanced type of metabolism with good qualities from both sides.

Striking a balance between sympathetic and parasympathetic is not all that is desirable. It is also important to have a good, strong metabolism capable of utilizing raw materials with maximum efficiency. The vertical scale shows the scale from the exceptionally strong metabolizer Type 10 to the good metabolizer Type 8 to the poor sympathetic metabolizer Type 6 to the poor parasympathetic metabolizer Type 7 to the poor balanced metabolizer Type 9 to the poorest metabolizer of all, Type 3. The Type 3 metabolizer only assimilates about 10% of what is eaten.

Chapter Nine

Physiological Reactions

Reactions to Eating and taking supplements will occur according to your metabolic type. As you follow...

As you follow a properly balanced nutritional program, changes begin to happen within your body. Often these changes are alarming and not at all what you expected.

Ideal Reaction

The ideal reaction is the gradual development of an increased "sense of well-being." At first you will notice you do not tire so easily. You "last" longer during the day, and you do not become tired so early in the evening. Next, you find you are not so tired in the mornings. You look forward to the new day and may awaken earlier. As your sense of well-being increases, you begin to feel more emotionally and psychologically secure. Little things do not bother you as they once did. Your old habit patterns begin to change from "grumpy" ones to "happy" ones.

Adverse

The ideal reaction often occurs, but more frequently there is a multitude of uncomfortable reactions, which normally come first, as your body chemistry begins to change. These reactions should not alarm you or cause undue apprehension. Any one or all of the following reactions may occur:

Toxic

After about two or three of weeks eating and taking supplements according to your metabolic type, it is normal to experience toxic reactions. You will gradually lose your appetite, become nauseated and may even develop a "toxic headache." Occasionally, you may also experience swelling in the various lymph glands throughout your body. The normal cells cleaning debris from the system faster than the liver, kidneys, skin and lungs can remove them from the body bring about these toxic reactions. At this point you can do two things to help:

• Discontinue the supplements for no more than a 5-day period. Continue the supplements again for 10 to 25 days. This cycle of 5 days off and 10 or more days on may have to be repeated several times, depending upon the depleted condition of your body and the amount of repair which is needed at the cellular level.

• Take a coffee enema to stimulate the excretion of toxins. The enema procedure is explained in Chapter IV. One or two a day may be taken depending upon the severity of the toxic condition. In an extreme toxic reaction both the discontinuance of supplements and the coffee enema should be used.

Allergic Reactions

Sometimes you may experience an allergic reaction; this is particularly true when the hydrochloric acid in the stomach is deficient and/or when the liver and adrenal glands are in a state of dysfunction or extreme exhaustion. The allergic reaction is similar to the toxic condition. You may just not feel well, be nauseated and/or even develop a skin rash, shortness of breath, etc. Taking too many supplements at once for the first time can bring about this reaction. If you tend to be allergic, you should start your supplemental program by taking only one supplement for 3 days, than adding the second one. Continue both for 3 more days, then add the third supplement. In 3 days add the next one and so forth, until you can tolerate the complete suggested supplemental program.

Physiological Balancing

As you begin to physiologically balance your body chemistry, other reactions may take place. It is not easy to change from lifelong habits of faulty eating of devitalized, processed foods to a new system of eating natural, life-giving foods and taking individualized needed supplements.

Following this metabolic program should bring about a readjustment of body chemistry. The body, meeting this changing situation, often responds in surprising ways to this process. The longer the deficiencies have existed, the more prevalent the response is likely to be. Additional reactions may occur as the body adapts and stabilizes. The reactions that often occur are:

- Canker sores
- Constipation
- Craving for unusual foods
- Diarrhea
- Dizziness
- Dry mouth
- Excessive gas
- Fever blisters
- Headaches
- Increased thirst
- Insomnia
- Loss of appetite
- Migrating pains
- Nausea
- Nervousness
- Nightmares
- Rash or hives
- Running nose
- Various body aches and pains, both in the joints and muscles
- Weakness

When these reactions occur, you can be assured your body is responding and changes are taking place. If you think of these as correcting crises, it will be easy to accept them as steps on the road to better health. If they occur, they are only temporary and are but a small price to pay for the long-lasting benefits.

Chapter Ten

Cancer Heroes' Testimonials

It is the nature of the medical Establishment to claim, "These cancer cases did not have cancer and that is why they are still alive and cancer-free." However, many of these patients were diagnosed by biopsy at the most prestigious institutions in the United States and Canada. Furthermore, in 1985, the actual biopsy slides were reviewed and confirmed by the renowned pathologist, Dr. Robert A. Good, Ph.D., former President of the Memorial Sloan-Kettering Cancer Center of New York City.

The Medical Establishment often accuses their enemy of doing exactly what they themselves do: Lie, deceive, and cover up. The media then screams it so loud and long that many of the gullible finally believe it to be true without any proof whatsoever. However, in the case of my patients, the Establishment cannot do this. This frustrates them to no end, and they have devised many ways to destroy and discredit the Cancer Heroes. Nowhere in the orthodox or alternative medical communities are so many Cancer Heroes truly documented with such long Cancer-free life spans.

Introduction to Dr. Kelley's Cancer Heroes

We are bringing to your attention two groups of cancer heroes. These cancer heroes, except as noted, were all alive and well and cancer-free in 1986. I unpluged my computer on the 30th of August, 1986, and closed the doors on the Kelley Program. Many of these heroes are still alive and well. I spoke to several in 1999 and 2000. I feel many others will contact me when they find this book. The Cancer Heroes are listed in two groups as follows:

Group I

Dr. Carol A. Morrison, M.D., F.A.C.C. and Dr. Kelley contacted these patients in late 1990. The following Group I patients were included in the 1982 edition of Metabolic Ecology by Fred Rohé. Many in this group of patients written up by Fred Rohé were copied and used by Nick Gonzalez for technical publication. Under the direction of the former president of Sloan-Kettering Institute, Dr. Robert Good, Mr. Gonzalez spent five years of serious investigation and review of the medical records of Dr. Kelley's patients. Of the thousands of cancer patients available, they narrowed the group down to 1,000 original patients who could meet the high standards of this study. Of the 1,000 qualified patients, mamy of the "Rohé 50" were used and written up. The 50 patients represented 25 types of cancer, half of which were diagnosed at major medical centers such as the Mayo Clinic, Sloan-Kettering Institute and others. The results of this study were extroadinary.

Hodgkin's Disease

Hodgkin's disease is a moderately rare cancer of the lymphocyte system and associated organs that claimed 1,500 lives in 1987.

Physicians have classified (in the claimed 1,500) this malignancy system of four "stages" (I-IV). Stage I represents early, localized disease; stage IV defines advanced, widely disseminated cancer involving many organs of the body. Stages II and III include more intermediate forms. Physicians further categorize Hodgkin's disease by the letters "A" and "B." The designation "A" refers to patients without symptoms. The letter "B" identifies patients with symptoms such as fevers, chills, night sweats, and fatigue. Hodgkin's, if untreated, is often rapidly fatal. "A single series of untreated patients reported by Croft in 1941," writes Devita, head of the National Cancer Institute, "leads us to believe that the course of patients with Hodgkin's disease, if left untreated, regardless of the stage, is brief, measured in 1 to 2 years. In that series, the median survival was less than 1 year and most patients were dead by year 2, with fewer than 5% alive after 5 years." At present, the "MOPP" chemotherapy regimen is the most widely recommended treatment for Hodgkin's. This protocol employs four drugs — nitrogen mustard, Oncovin (vincristine), procarbazine and prednisone — given once every 28 days for at 6 months. As Devita explains, "Unless chemotherapy is contraindicated for medical reasons, all patients treated with MOPP and other combinations should be given a minimum of 6 cycles (a dose) or as many cycles as needed to achieve a complete remission, plus additional cycles to consolidate the remission."(1) With protocols such as this, at least 50% of all patients will survive 5 years.

Michael Moreland

Michael Moreland is a 37-year old man from Washington State alive 9 years since diagnosed with Hodgkin's disease. In late 1977, Moreland developed mild fatigue and a tender swelling in his neck that rapidly increased in size. In January of 1978 he consulted his family physician, who suspected a low-grade infection and prescribed a course of penicillin therapy. With treatment, the swelling did decrease slightly over a period of a week, but then worsened. In addition, Moreland began experiencing drenching night sweats as well as sharp pain in the upper part of his chest. Several weeks later, Moreland returned to his physician. A chest X-ray revealed a large upper mediastinal mass, and laboratory studies were significant for an elevated white blood count of 21,000 (upper limit of normal 10,000). Because of these findings, on February 6, 1978 Moreland entered Vancouver Memorial Hospital in Vancouver, Washington. On admission, Moreland was noted to have extensive lymphadenopathy in the cervical area, described in the records as: "A very large mass present in the left side of the neck with some surrounding smaller masses also present. There are some more discrete masses on the right side as well, measuring up to 3 to 4 centimeters in diameter. There is a bilateral auxiliary adenopathy present." The following day, Moreland went to surgery. Subsequent evaluation of the tissue specimen confirmed an aggressive form of Hodgkin's disease, well-described in the official pathology report: "There is no question that nodules are being formed in this lymph node but in many areas the picture is more than a mixed cellularity type and there are remarkably large collections composed mainly of malignant reticulohitiocytic cells with lymphocyte depletion." With a diagnosis of Hodgkin's confirmed Moreland was readmitted to Vancouver Memorial on February 13 for additional tests. A chest X-ray showed:

"Mediastinal adenopathy which is a little more pronounced on the right. There is evidence of bilateral cervical nodes." A lymphangiogram, a dye study of the abdominal lymph node system, demonstrated extensive disease, as summarized in the records: "Abnormal lymphangiogram due to enlarged nodes caused by Hodgkin's disease at L2, L3 and probably along the right iliac chain."

On February 13, Moreland underwent a staging laparotomy — exploratory abdominal surgery — and removal of his spleen, a procedure often performed in patients with Hodgkin's. Although the spleen was free of disease, a periaortic influenced lymph node was positive for cancer. At the same time a bone marrow biopsy was attempted, but the specimen could not be conclusively analyzed. Moreland was told he suffered advanced Hodgkin's disease, officially recorded as: "Hodgkin's disease, nodular sclerosed type, stage IIIB." His doctors advised that aggressive multi-agent chemotherapy was the only hope for prolonged survival and proposed their standard 6-month, 6-cycle course of MOPP. Moreland agreed to the treatment, which he began in late February as an outpatient at the Vancouver Clinic.

After the first round of drugs Moreland became extremely weak, fatigued, and anorexic. His symptoms did improve over a 2-week period, but while undergoing the second cycle, Moreland became severely ill. He did struggle through a third course, but felt so debilitated, decided to discontinue chemotherapy. The attending physician warned Moreland that without appropriate treatment, he would quickly die, and suggested a 6-month course of radiation as an alternative. Moreland accepted the plan and in late May received his first dose of cobalt to the chest.

Once again Moreland became ill, and in mid-July, after receiving a total of 4060 rads to the chest and upper abdomen, Moreland refused further treatment. At the same time, he was not believed to be cancer-free. According to Moreland his doctors warned that he would die within a year, unless he agreed to additional therapy.

Moreland did not change his mind. Instead, after investigating alternative approaches to cancer, he met with Dr. Kelley in late July and shortly thereafter began the Kelley Program. Within a month he noticed improved energy and well-being and within a year, says he felt better than he had for a decade.

Moreland followed the full regimen for 3 years, and today, 9 years since his diagnosis, he remains in excellent health. He also has two healthy children, currently, aged 4 and 6; this is unusual, since MOPP chemotherapy causes sterility in a majority of male patients. Despite his abbreviated courses of both chemotherapy and radiation I believe Moreland is a relatively simple case to evaluate. Although there are, in the medical literature, several documented instances of patients with advanced Hodgkin's enjoying prolonged survival after incomplete treatment with MOPP, such cases are extremely rare. While he did undergo radiotherapy, all of it was directed to his chest and upper abdomen. His extensive lower abdominal and pelvic tumors were never irradiated.

In summary, Moreland suffered Stage IIIB Hodgkin's disease, treated with partial courses of chemotherapy and radiation. When first seen by Dr. Kelley, he was clinically debilitated and not, according to his doctors, in remission; it seems reasonable to attribute this patient's prolonged survival and current good health to his nutritional protocol.

Scott Stirling

Scott Stirling is a 53-year-old Canadian, alive 27 years since developing Hodgkin's disease. In January of 1971, Stirling noticed a swelling on the left side of his neck.

He consulted his local physician who believed the lesion to be a benign cyst, and no additional evaluation was recommended.

Over the following year, the swelling fluctuated in size. Finally, when his neck enlarged dramatically in June of 1972, Stirling returned to his doctor, and was admitted to Reddy Memorial Hospital in Toronto. Stirling subsequently went to surgery for removal of the presumed cyst. However, the mass proved to be a matted collection of cancerous lymph nodes, 15 of which were found positive for nodular sclerosing Hodgkin's disease.

Stirling was transferred to Princess Margaret Hospital for further study and treatment. Serial X-rays of the mediastinum (mid-chest) showed no evidence of metastatic disease, but additional X-rays confirmed extension of cancer throughout the pelvis, described in the radiology report as ". . . filling defects and dilated intranodal and peripheral sinusoids in the paraortic nodes on the left. These changes are typical of early involvement by Hodgkin's disease."

A bone scan demonstrated abnormalities in the pelvic region consistent with metastases, summarized as: "Increased deposition of activity in the left side of the pelvis and the left sacroiliac joint. Appearance suggests the possibility of an abnormality of this site."

A liver-spleen scan revealed an enlarged spleen, and a liver infiltrated with tumor. The records describe: "Appearances on the anterior and right lateral scans are strongly suggestive of the presence of a space-occupying lesion located in the anterior right lobe (of the liver) — There is also poor concentration of activity within the left lobe, suggesting the presence of an extensive infiltrating lesion. The spleen is moderately enlarged."

The standard 6-month, 6-cycle MOPP chemotherapy protocol was recommended. After agreeing to the treatment plan, Stirling received his first round of MOPP as an inpatient on June 30, 1972. He tolerated the chemotherapy without significant side effects and was discharged from the hospital in early July. But after the second course of drugs Stirling developed severe weakness, fatigue and anorexia. He did eventually recover, and returned to the hospital for a third round of MOPP in late August. While being treated, Stirling again became very ill and insisted the chemotherapy be stopped. At the time of discharge several days later, he was told he most probably would not live a year.

Stirling then began a long automobile trip through the United States. In September of 1972, while staying with friends in Arizona, he quite by chance learned of Dr. Kelley's work. Several days later he was on the road again, heading for Dallas and an appointment with Dr. Kelley. Within a week, Stirling had begun the full Kelley regimen.

Shortly after, the lymph nodes in his neck and auxiliary regions suddenly enlarged, within a period of months, the swelling regressed, and today, 27 years after his diagnosis, he still follows the Kelley Program, remains cancer-free and is in excellent health. Although a single course of MOPP can cause sterility, Stirling now has two children of his own and a third by marriage.

In summary, Stirling suffered widely metastatic, stage IV Hodgkin's disease. After an abbreviated course of MOPP, the disease recurred explosively. However, Stirling's cancer went into remission, apparently for good, as he pursued only the Kelley Program. Update December 1998; Scott and family are doing fine, cancer-free, healthy and happy in San Diego.

Lung Cancer

Philip Bonfiglio

Philip Bonfiglio is a 52-year-old man from Ohio, who has survived 13 years since his diagnosis of metastatic squamous cell carcinoma of the lung.

In early 1974 Bonfiglio, a heavy smoker, developed a persistent upper respiratory infection and cough. He consulted his family doctor, who prescribed a course of antibiotic therapy. Despite the treatment, the symptoms only worsened, and in March Mr. Bonfiglio returned to his physician. At that time a chest X-ray revealed a 3-centimeter (cm) mass in the upper lobe of the right lung.

Bonfiglio was admitted to Akron City Hospital on April 7, 1974, and the following day went for exploratory chest surgery. He was found to have a large inoperable tumor in the right lung that had metastasized to many lymph nodes. These findings are clearly described in the operative note: "A tumor approximately 4 cm in greatest diameter was found in the periphery of the posterior segment of the right upper lobe (of the lung). In the area below the azygos vein were multiple nodes, which extended posteriorly up along the vena cave and acquired a maximum diameter of about 3.5-cm. Because of the massive involvement of the mediastinum, curative resection was not feasible."

Evaluation of a biopsy specimen confirmed: "Poorly differentiated carcinoma consistent with squamous cell type." In addition, all lymph nodes removed at surgery were positive for metastatic disease.

Bonfiglio's doctors recommended a course of cobalt radiation treatment, which he began while still hospitalized. Nevertheless, he was told that even with such treatment, his chances of surviving one year were dim.

In the discharge summary, the attending physician wrote: ". . . The patient, due to the metastatic nature of this carcinoma, does have a poor prognosis."

Bonfiglio completed the suggested regimen of 5,000 rads to the lungs as an outpatient. When the tumors continued to grow despite the radiation, a course of intensive chemotherapy was proposed. But since his disease was believed incurable, Bonfiglio refused all further orthodox treatment. Instead, he decided to investigate unconventional cancer therapies and soon learned of Dr. Kelley, consulted with him and began the Kelley Program in late spring.

Over a several-month period, his persistent respiratory symptoms resolved, and within a year, Bonfiglio says he felt better than he had for a decade.

Today, 13 years after his diagnosis, Bonfiglio still follows his nutritional protocol and is in excellent health with no sign of his once-metastatic disease.

Squamous cell carcinoma of the lung is one of the most deadly of cancers. The 5-year survival rate for patients with Stage III disease, regardless of treatment, is less than 5%.(1) Stanley reports a median survival of only 24-27 weeks in 32 symptomatic patients, such as Bonfiglio, with unresectable tumors (2).

In summary, Bonfiglio suffered inoperable, mestastatic lung cancer, which did not respond to a course of cobalt therapy.

It therefore seems appropriate to attribute this patient's long-term survival to the Kelley Program.

References:

1. Devita, V.T., et al. Cancer — Principles and Practice of Oncology. **Philadelphia; J.B. Lippincott Company, 1982, page 409.**

2. Stanley, K.E. "Prognostic Factors for Survival in Patients with Inoperable Lung Cancer." Journal of the National Cancer Institute, **65:25-32, 1980.**

Colon Cancer

Robert Beesley

Mr. Robert Beesley is a 67-year-old man from Iowa who has survived nearly 12 years since his diagnosis of metastatic colon cancer.

In mid-1975, Beesley first became fatigued and developed severe constipation alternating with episodes of watery diarrhea. Some months later, after noticing bright red blood in his stool, he consulted his family physician who referred him for tests at a local clinic. At that time, a barium enema revealed a large, 5.7-cm. mass in the right colon, which was believed to be consistent with cancer.

On July 7, 1975, Beesley was admitted to Iowa Methodist Medical Center for further evaluation. A liver-spleen scan was positive for a "suspicious defect of the left lobe of the liver" that measured approximately 2.5 centimeters in diameter.

Other studies, however, including chest X-rays, showed no sign of metastatic disease. The following day Beesley went to surgery for removal of the right half of his large intestine.

In addition to the colon tumor, he was found to have unresectable metastases in both lobes of the liver, described in the operative note as "two lesions in the liver, one in the right and one in the left lobe of the liver." The right lesion was larger than the left, measuring about 2 by 2 cms.

Review of the specimen confirmed a fulminant grade III Adenocarcinoma extending into the adjacent tissues, as described in the formal pathology report: The rectal pouch is filled with bulky ulcerated neoplasm, which is almost completely circumferential measuring 10 by 6 by 2 cm. Tumor infiltrates directly into the contiguous mesentery (the tissues adjacent to the large intestine)" — Beesley was told he might live 3 to 6 months, at most.

The attending physicians, believing him beyond cure, recommended neither chemotherapy nor radiation.

After leaving the hospital on July 21, 1975, Beesley decided to investigate unorthodox approaches to cancer. Later that summer, he learned of Dr. Kelley, consulted with him and began the Kelley Program. Beesley continued the full Kelley regimen for 7 years before tapering down to a maintenance program, which he still follows. Today, despite the initial terminal prognosis, he is in excellent health and cancer-free. Although he has not been formally evaluated since his original surgery 12 years ago, Beesley believes his continued survival is proof enough of his cure. Colon cancer, when metastatic to the liver, is invariably rapidly fatal.

Pestana and colleagues at the Mayo Clinic report a mean survival of only 9.0 months in 353 patients presented with liver involvement.(1)

In similar studies, Bengmark describes an average survival of only 7.8 months(2), and Morris a median survival of 11.4 months.(3)

Obviously, Mr. Beesley's progress represents a most unusual outcome for this disease.

As a footnote to this case, the author was surprised to learn that supporters of Lawrence Burton, an unconventional therapist with a clinic in the Bahamas, had been advertising Mr. Beesley as a "Burton Success." When I mentioned these reports to Mr. Beesley, he explained that he received several weeks of Burton Therapy in the fall of 1975 — after he had already improved significantly on the Kelley program.

Furthermore, Mr. Beesley claims he never finished the prescribed Burton protocol, and never received any further treatment from Burton. Mr. Beesley himself attributes his recovery to his many years on the Kelley regimen and not to Burton.

Unfortunately, I have found over the years that many unorthodox therapists repeatedly claim Dr. Kelley's long-term patients as their own; misrepresentation obviously does not help cancer patients.

References:

1. Pestana, C., et al. **"The Natural History of Carcinoma of the Colon and Rectum."** American Journal of Surgery, **108:826-829, 1964**

2. Bengmark, S., and Hafstrom, L. **"The Natural History of Primary and Secondary Malignant Tumors of the Liver."** Cancer, **23:198-202, 1969**

3. Morris, M.J., et al. **"Hepatic Metastases from Colorectal Carcinoma."** Australia & New Zealand Journal of Surgery, **47:365-368, 1977.**

Breast Cancer

Sonia Nemethy

Sonia Nemethy is a 53-year-old woman alive more than 17 years since diagnosed with breast carcinoma.

Nemethy first noticed a painless mass in her right breast in 1970. After biopsy studies confirmed infiltrating carcinoma, she went to surgery for a right radical mastectomy at St. Anthony's hospital in Florida.

Nemethy was believed cured and received no further treatment at that time. In 1973, after a second tumor developed in the left breast, Mrs. Namethy returned to St. Anthony's and underwent a left radical mastectomy for what proved to be infiltrating carcinoma.

Nemethy was again assumed to be cured, but over the following year, her health gradually deteriorated. She suffered fatigue, lethargy and bouts of depression persisting for months at a time.

In mid-1974 Nemethy also developed pain along the length of the vertebral column and into the right shoulder.

By late 1974 the pain was so severe at times she was unable to dress or walk. Although Nemethy consulted her physicians repeatedly, an evaluation was not pursued. Finally, in May of 1975, at Mrs. Nemethy's insistence, her doctor arranged for a series of spinal X-rays. These studies revealed an obvious abnormality in the fifth lumbar segment, described as "indicative of osteolytic metastasis disease."

On May 28, 1975, Mrs. Nemethy returned to surgery for a bilateral oophorectomy (removal of both ovaries), a procedure doctors hoped would slow the growth of the tumor and ease her bone pain. Despite the surgery, Nemethy was told she probably would not live out the year.

In desperation, after leaving the hospital on May 31, Nemethy decided to investigate alternative cancer therapies.

She quickly learned of Dr. Kelley, consulted with him and began the Kelley Program in the summer of 1975.

Within 6 months, the persistent pain and depression completely resolved. Furthermore, a bone scan performed at the end 1975 showed some improvement, and a third bone scan from mid-1976, was completely normal.

Today, 12 years after her last episode with cancer, Nemethy still follows the Kelley Program and is in excellent condition.

As discussed previously, the 5-year survival rate (at that time) for patients with metastatic breast cancer approaches 0% regardless of therapy. And oophorectomy (removal of ovary) which may lead to symptomatic improvement in this group, is not curative. As Hellman writes, "In patients whose tumors are estrogen-dependent the procedure can be expected to induce a regression lasting 9 months to 12 months. In unselected series (of patients) almost 30% to 40% of patients will respond. Prophylactic castration (ovary removal) following mastectomy does not decrease the potential relapse rate or prolong the survival of those who relapse."(1)

In summary, this patient developed evidence of metastases after successive mastectomies for recurring breast carcinoma. Although she did undergo oophorectomy, Nemethy continued to deteriorate after the procedure. Her extensive disease and many symptoms resolved only after she began the Kelley Program.

References:

1. Devita, V.T., et al. Cancer — Principles and Practice of Oncology, **Philadelphia; J.B. Lippincott Company, 1982, page 945.**

Stomach Cancer

Elizabeth Wojt

Elizabeth Wojt is a 47-year-old woman from New Jersey, alive 10 years since her diagnosis of stomach carcinoma.

Before her bout with cancer Wojt had a long history of general poor health and chronic digestive problems. In 1974 she first experienced episodes of severe abdominal pain that usually occurred between meals and were relieved by eating. Over the following three years her symptoms gradually worsened, although she was not normally evaluated until spring of 1977. At that time a barium swallow revealed a tumor, described in an official report as "suspicious lesion in the fundus and cardiac of the stomach."

Wojt was referred to a gastroenterologist, who biopsied the suspect tissue during endoscopy (examination of the stomach with a flexible tube inserted down the esophagus). After review, the specimen was identified as a carcinoma.

Wojt was admitted to Patterson General Hospital on April 17 and the following day, she went to surgery (for a radical subtotal gastrectomy, which is resection of most of the stomach). The tumor had already metastasized into the surrounding tissues and lymph nodes; the final pathology report describes: "Adenocarcinoma of the stomach with metastases to the gastrocolic nodes and omentum."

Wojt was told she most likely would not live a year. Nevertheless, after leaving Patterson Hospital in late April, she was referred to the Memorial Sloan-Kettering Cancer Center in New York for possible experimental treatment. But Wojt, who already knew of Dr. Kelley's work, decided to refuse all orthodox therapy. Instead, that same month she consulted Dr. Kelley and began the full Kelley Program. Wojt followed her nutritional regimen for 5 years. At present, 10 years after her diagnosis, she is in excellent health apparently cured of her once-metastatic disease. According to Wojt, her doctors are "dumbfounded" by her prolonged survival.

Wojt is indeed a remarkable case. The 5-year survival rate for patients with metastatic stomach cancer is close to zero — even with aggressive therapy. Wojt received neither chemotherapy nor radiation after her surgery, and chose to follow only the Kelley Program.

Group II

Group II consists of patients' stories collected and written up in 1982 by Fred Rohé for his book *Metabolic Ecology.* Stories are presented in the patients' own words and include Dr. Kelley's spontaneous thoughts recorded immediately upon reading them. Rohé selected 24 patients of the thousands available. For this booklet we have presented 11 of these for your review.

Leukemia

Thomas M., Alexandria, LA

5-Year Victory over Leukemia

At age 61, this lawyer, blessed with a lovely wife and 8 children, was diagnosed at Ochsner Clinic, New Orleans, as having acute myelogenous spinal leukemia.

My friends at Ochsner Clinic opined that the condition was terminal and that I had at best a few months and at worst a few days to live.

"Following three courses of Cytosar and Thiogunine at the Clinic (from October 7, 1977 through about mid-December 1977), I fortunately had a remission. I was to continue with maintenance therapy,

which the medics told me would, at best, improve the quality of life. There was slim, if any, hope for recovery.

Dr. Kelley's book miraculously came to my wife's attention. We visited him in Washington in December 1977. We were enthusiastic, and I got on the program and experienced dramatic improvement. The idea that you treat the body, or host, and not the symptoms was so intellectually stimulating and sensible, I wondered why my medical friends and my doctor son could not understand and why they discouraged and belittled my efforts. I shortly resumed my practice, golf and a normal but different lifestyle.

About midsummer of 1978 it became apparent that to continue the chemotherapy would destroy any hope I had of bodybuilding. These shots nauseated disrupted me and knocked my blood count from near normal to complete disarray. My mind indicated that they be discontinued, despite advice to the contrary.

I've continued with Metabolic Medicine and on the complete lifestyle change that holistic medicine demands for optimum health. I've no problems with leukemia since the initial remission was obtained. I know that when I took the chemo maintenance, my body was disrupted. I know that when it was discontinued, I continued to improve without the disruption of the blood picture and the nausea.

Metabolic Medicine is so sensible, it's hard to see why anyone could dispute that it has a place in the lives of the acutely ill. Nothing's perfect and nothing makes one eternal, but in my case, I'm thankful for the opportunity for the benefits of this non-toxic therapy and the miracle it brought for me. Some call my luck 'spontaneous remission'; maybe so, I believe that Metabolic Medicine makes for "spontaneous remissions" from the symptoms of terminal illness in those whose bodies have not been abused beyond repair, whether by neglect or over treatment.

Some call such letters 'testimonials' instead of 'case histories.' For me, this is a very brief history of my case for whatever value and hope it may give to others.

One last observation ought to be made. Some decry holistic therapy that of 'hucksters' and 'quacks.' Most practitioners of this art (and there are many medical men in this kind of practice) are those who have had a terminal diagnosis for themselves or loved ones and were disenchanted by the hopelessness and horror of traditional therapies. I've met many of the 'greats.' None that I know drive Mercedes. All are healers and not moneymakers. The cost of a year of holistic medicine for me doesn't exceed the cost of one week of treatment in any good conventional cancer hospital.

I enjoy my family, my practice and my life. I'm grateful for a therapy that has, thus for, worked for me."

Dr. Kelley: My dear friend Tom brings up a lot of wonderful memories and brings to mind the subject of soft tumor. Soft tumors, it should be emphasized, are an entirely different condition from what we normally think of as cancer. What are soft tumors? I classify the leukemias, lymphomas, melanomas, tumors of the immune system, and those of the blood system as soft tumors. It is very frightening that soft tumors are becoming so prevalent in children. Before 1979 we find that the highest cause of death in children was traumatic accidents, such as falling out of a tree or running in front of a car. But since 1979 we find that the leading cause of death of children under 16 is cancer, a sad commentary on our society. Most of these cancer deaths are from soft tumors.

Tom was a patient 62 years of age. A lot of people, as they get older, as their immune systems malfunction, as their energies wane, as they become exhausted, develop soft tumors. Tom was a professional person who had a hard, active life and developed leukemia; it was very, very severe, in fact, so bad that he'd started collecting fluid in the abdomen, a condition that's always fatal. It was quite rewarding to have a person with this condition so willing to give 100% attention and effort to following Metabolic Medicine in such a severe, advanced disease. It's always a joy to me to see a patient so conscientious and pure of heart in following the program. In Tom's case we find that the side effects of the program — such as resuming his law practice and feeling terrific — were also quite astounding.

Breast Cancer

Judy S., Glendale, CA

9-Year Victory over Breast Cancer

"In January of 1973 I had another checkup from my breast doctor in Beverly Hills (a breast surgeon, tops in this field). I'd been going to him every 6 months for 2 years, then every 4 months for 1 year, then every 2 months until January of 1973. At that time he told me the lump in my left breast had gotten very large and I'd have to go to surgery. His nurse told me he was an expert and that he could tell by feeling the lump if it was malignant or benign and that a mammogram gave a 96% account of the tumor whether it was malignant or benign. The doctor explained how carefully he would remove the breast, and about bras for women whose breasts have been removed. He also was going to Europe for two months; my surgery would be scheduled when he returned.

I had read Dr. Kelley's book some months before and decided to go to one of our local health food stores where I'd bought the book to talk to the owner, who was always well- informed on natural foods and vitamins. She told me to call some people in town who'd gone to Dr. Kelley and that I should by all means go to him. I was encouraged when I talked to the people who'd gone to Dr. Kelley. All had cancer at one time, and one person in particular was most helpful to me.

I was just starting a new job at this time as a singer in a famous Italian restaurant doing opera and musical comedy. This was several times around for me to 'start' my career again after having three children and being a housewife for a few years. I was excited, but was feeling good.

I flew to see Dr. Kelley, then in Texas, and my cancer count was 600. I took Dr. Kelley's advice, went home and started on his program of diet, enemas and supplements. I was weak at first but in a few months, really started feeling so much better. My husband was totally against the program. My friends at church thought I was crazy, and I found it was difficult to pay for all the supplements, but was determined to stay on the entire program.

I kept my appointment with the breast surgeon but had been on Dr. Kelley's program for two months when I returned for my examination. I was told the lump had gone down and no surgery was needed. I left his office in early March of 1973 and haven't been back since. The following year I was not only singing four nights a week but was working at a busy TV station 8 hours per day.

I continued to see Dr. Kelley once a year. My cancer count continued to decrease until my last checkup in August of 1977 when my cancer count was 60, which Dr. Kelley says is normal.

I can't say enough about how I'd never take any other treatment for cancer than Dr. Kelley's. In fact, I consult him on all my physical problems, I wouldn't think of taking another doctor's advice without asking Dr. Kelley's first. I tell everyone about Dr. Kelley!

I'm a most happy and satisfied patient of Dr. Kelley!"

Dr. Kelley: **"Many people want me to make decisions for them: Should I have chemotherapy? Should I do this? Should I do that? Should I do what the doctor tells me to do, or not to do what he tells me to do? These kinds of questions have given me many, many hours of frustration and anxiety. First of all, I'm in a legal position where I can't tell the patient not to do what the doctor tells them to do. And I know the physician does the very best he knows how. It's just that he's suffering from a great deal of ignorance. So, legally I'm in a very bad situation.**

Morally, I'm in even a worse position. It becomes quite a dilemma in my mind. All of us would like to take the easy way out and have somebody make our decisions for us. But that doesn't give us the education we need and the experiences that are our responsibility to take on.

"So, the way I address the problem is this: God's given us a rulebook to follow for our education. He tells us these are the principles we should follow in our life's activities; and if we do these things, this will happen; and if we do those things, that will happen. And then He lets us have the total freedom and free will to do what we will, and live with the consequences. I study and try to find the basic principles.

In a similar sense, Metabolic Medicine is essentially a program based upon what I've observed in thousands of cases to be sound principles. I'm continually improving my understanding of these principles and all I can do is educate the patient to the best of my ability. I look at each patient and say, 'These are the things that I've observed, and these are the principles upon which our program exists.'

If you have a life threatening situation, such as a tumor mass blocking the colon or blocking the bladder, the stomach, or the air passage, you should, of course, address it in such a way as to take care of it. Orthodox medicine has done an excellent job of addressing life-threatening situations such as trauma, and infections. Each individual patient must make the decision in a life-threatening situation. If you have a 5-lb. tumor in the abdomen and it's dead from your doing a nutritional program, it's certainly going to be easier to remove this 5-lb. tumor and throw it away than it would be to sit there and have your immune system and body chemistry gradually dissolve it, using a lot of energy and stressing the body to dissolve it into the bloodstream and then cleaning out the bloodstream through the liver and the other organs of elimination.

In any situation that's addressed, you must to hold to basic principles and do some ecological thinking. I'd be stupid to say you're going to follow a nutritional program when a tumor's blocking the intestinal tract and you can't get any food into your body and can't get any nutritional support. It'd likewise be stupid to say,

'I'm going to take chemotherapy because I have a snarled tumor in my colon and I'll take chemotherapy to the point of death and then have a better chance of survival.' Every situation is addressed individually, with understanding, knowledge and wisdom."

Breast and Liver Cancer

Rosswitha A., Malaga, Spain

6-Year Victory over Breast and Liver Cancer

At the time of writing this testimonial, Rosswitha had a 4-year victory over breast and liver cancer. Nutritional Counseling Service heard from her in 1983, and she was in excellent health and enthusiastic about the program.

"*In June 1976, I discovered a lump on my left breast. My gynecologist sent me to have a mammography done. The result was positive and he told me it was almost certainly a malignant growth. I went to a surgeon who examined me thoroughly and had some more X-rays done. He found I had an enlarged liver and said he'd have to do an exploratory operation before doing a mastectomy. After the operation he told me I had cancer on the liver, too, and that there was no point in removing the breast. He said he'd give me two sessions of chemotherapy. I decided (after two weeks of pills and injections) to go to the University Clinic Hospital in Frankfurt, Germany, where my parents live. The surgeon in Malaga, Spain, gave me a report to take to Germany, which said I had cancer of the breast with a massive growth on the liver and another in the abdominal area.*

I had more examinations and a scan test in Frankfurt. The surgeon there confirmed the Spanish report and said the growth of the tumor was fist-size. He told my husband and myself there was no cure and the most we could hope for was a remission. He'd not say how long a remission. He advised me to have a mastectomy to remove the primary growth in the breast and to have the ovaries taken out to change the hormone balance in the body, which would make the subsequent chemotherapy treatment more effective.

We were given the impression that there was no time to lose and few alternatives. I decided to have the surgery and chemotherapy in the hope that it'd give me a remission and enough time to seek a cure elsewhere. By this time I was feeling bad, suffering, I think, from the reactions of the chemotherapy in Spain. I had an infection in the bladder, which was painful. My hair was beginning to fall out. I felt weak and depressed. When I returned to the hospital a few days later for the operation, I could hardly walk. I was operated on July 28 and started chemotherapy (injections) on September 1.

I stayed in the hospital only three days after each chemotherapy treatment, and, after the third session, the doctors began to comment on this, comparing me with the other patients, who were on their backs for days after the treatments. I suggested it could be due to the diet I was on. The moment I learned of my cancer, I had put myself on a healthy diet, cut all the chemicalized foods and made adjustments to it when a friend in Germany gave a book on food for cancer patients. The doctors and nurses seemed amused at this and said I could eat anything I wanted — it'd make no difference. I continued with my diet.

A woman doctor in the chemotherapy ward seemed more willing than the others to discuss my problem with me. I told her of my intention to seek a cure and showed her a booklet on Dr. Nieper of Hanover. She'd not heard of Dr. Nieper or his treatment. She told me I was responding well to the chemotherapy and should forget about any other kind of treatment until I had completed the chemotherapy sessions. I couldn't forget about it, though, as I was becoming more convinced that chemotherapy was not going to give me the long remission I'd hoped for and that I'd better look quickly for an alternative treatment.

When told I had cancer, my husband and I did the contrary to what many people do in this situation; We told everyone we knew about my problem, hoping somebody could point us to a cure. My husband, publishing the English-language magazine on the Costa de Sol (an international retirement center full of informed people from all over the world), was in a good position to find out about things, and, even before I began chemotherapy in Frankfurt, we'd gathered a lot of information and were writing to a dozen doctors and clinics around Europe who were using unorthodox treatments to cure cancer. A friend gave us a copy of the Healthview Newsletter at this time. The long interview with Dr. Kelley, in which he explained very clearly his theory and treatment, gave me tremendous hope. Here was proof that cancer was being cured.

I was given a break in the chemotherapy treatment and returned to our home in Spain towards the end of November 1976. The chemotherapy was taking its toll, and I felt I was going downhill: bald, often depressed, very weak and in pain. Until then, even during the worst moments, I believed I'd somehow fight my way back to good health. When I read somewhere that only one in ten thousand survived chemotherapy, I assumed I was going to be the one in ten thousand. Now, I wasn't so sure, and was so weak, felt I couldn't go on. The cramps in my stomach became unbearable. We called in a local doctor, a friend of ours, and he gave me an injection to kill the pain. He called my husband aside and told him that he'd given me morphine and would come immediately any hour of the day or night to give me more, as needed. He thought I couldn't live many more days. Another doctor friend, who runs a local clinic where I was having regular blood checks, had received a report from the Frankfurt hospital, which stated I had a fist-sized growth on the liver and several other plum-size growths in the pelvis area. Questioned by my husband as to my chances, he simply shook his head and said, "Malo, malo, malo" (bad, bad, bad).

*I felt the stomach cramps were indigestion and became extremely careful about what I ate. In fact, at this point I was almost too frightened to eat anything. I knew now I had to do something quickly before it was too late. We began studying all the information we'd gathered on cancer cures and set ourselves a time limit of 2 days to make our decision. This was perhaps the most agonizing time of all. I felt we had to make the right choice the first time, as there wouldn't be time for another. My Yoga teacher joined us (I had started Yoga some weeks before and each day was doing some simple exercises, mainly breathing exercises, which I believed would strengthen me and help me relax). We had several books on cancer treatments but kept coming back to Dr. Kelley's **One Answer to Cancer.** It made sense to me and I was particularly impressed by the fact that Dr. Kelley had gone through what I was going through and had cured himself. I'd felt convinced about Dr. Kelley for weeks, but was put off by the distance I'd have to travel to see him. He seemed so far away and I dreaded the journey. I finally made my decision and phoned. The Kelley Foundation in Winthrop, Washington. As much as my husband wanted to go with me, we agreed that it'd be more practical if he stayed at home with our three small children (ages 5, 7, and 9) and I be accompanied on the journey by my yoga teacher, who — being American — would probably prove more useful during our time in the States.*

Winthrop was quite a contrast to the hospital in Frankfurt. I'd been very impressed at first by the vast buildings, the army of doctors and nurses, the apparent efficiency of the Frankfurt Hospital and felt, mistakenly, I'd come to the right place and that here they must be clever enough to cure anything. Arriving in Winthrop, I wondered if it could be possible that such important work as Dr. Kelley's was being carried out in such a tiny place miles and miles from anywhere.

Dr. Kelley himself was quite different from the doctors in Frankfurt who'd made me feel I was being a nuisance every time I asked a question about my condition and treatment. This attitude I found frustrating. My life was in their hands and I considered it was my a right to know exactly what they were doing with it. The other patients didn't seem to mind being treated like children who should keep quiet and do as they were told. At least, I never heard any ask questions about the treatment they were receiving or drugs they were being given. When I suggested to a fellow-patient receiving chemotherapy and in constant pain that she eat something healthier than Frankfurter sausages and ice cream, she said the doctors knew best and they'd surely not give her food that wasn't good for her.

At last I spoke with a doctor who treated me like an intelligent human being and was quite willing to discuss all the details of my illness. Dr. Kelley explained everything very clearly, admitted I was in a bad state but said he saw no reason why I shouldn't come through if I followed the treatment. It was largely up to me. I felt tremendous relief and hope. It was like the chance to live had been taken away and was now being given back to me. I now had a chance and that was all I asked for. If my recovery depended largely on my own efforts, I knew I'd succeed, as I was ready to do anything to get well.

"Returning home, I stopped off at Frankfurt where I had a mid-December appointment for more chemotherapy. I hated the idea of having more drugs pumped into me but relatives and friends at Frankfurt, nervous at the thought of my dropping the orthodox treatment, advised me to keep the appointment. Dr. Kelley didn't seem opposed to the idea of my having one more session. I went to the hospital but the moment they started giving me the injections, I felt I'd made a terrible mistake and that all the drugs were going to do was poison my body and weaken it even more.

I felt terrible afterwards. I was in bed for several days with pains, nausea and exhaustion, and felt depressed. I felt so weak I couldn't face the journey home to spend Christmas with my husband and my children. I spent all Christmas day vowing I'd take no more drugs. All I wanted now was to go home and start Dr. Kelley's program.

I began the nutritional program on January 3, 1977. Swallowing all the supplements and taking the morning enema was a bit of an effort at first but after a few days, I got used to this procedure and it became routine. I suffered none of the reactions Dr. Kelley warned me about. In fact, I began to feel better almost immediately. The pains went and, except for an ache in the shoulder during a bout of flu last winter, I've had none since I starting the program.

I followed Dr. Kelley's advice and became selfish for a few months, concentrating all my thought and efforts on my own health and helping my body to become strong again. I continued my daily yoga exercises, started a vegetable garden so we could have fresh vegetables and I began to make my own bread, from whole-grain flour we bought from an old mill in an inland Pueblo. I felt now I was doing something positive and, after months of pain and depression, was now on the road to recovery.

After eight months, I was re-tested and Dr. Kelley wrote me to tell me I was making very good progress. This was tremendously encouraging news, but I already knew in myself that I was getting stronger with each week that passed. Around this time, I went to see the surgeon in Malaga who'd examined me the previous year. He examined me and was amazed that he could no longer feel the *growth on the liver; he thought it had gone. I wondered whether he was trying to cheer me up but later learned through a mutual doctor friend that he discussed my case during a medical reunion in Malaga and said I was taking some weird treatment in America and, whatever it was, it seemed to be working.*

We have several doctor friends here in Spain who are familiar with my case. Whenever I see them, they seem very pleased to see how well I'm looking but neither show curiosity nor neither they express the slightest interest in the treatment I'm on. This puzzles me as I should have thought a doctor, more than any other person, would want to know how I'm recovering from an illness they regard as incurable and which, according to them, should've killed me more than a year before.

After a year of staying most of the time at home, concentrating quietly on the business of getting well and following my nutritional program to the letter, I began, little by little, to go out and become more active. I'm now leading a normal life. I run a home, am involved in the PTA at my children's Spanish school, and help my husband in the office three times a week. I might still have some cancer in my body but this does not worry me. I'm convinced it's only a matter of months before I'm completely cured. Dr. Kelley told me that my illness could turn out to be a blessing in disguise. I couldn't believe this at the time, but now I'm sure he was right. I feel I am starting a new life. My family is now eating a healthier diet. And I feel my illness has brought my husband and myself closer. I also have the added satisfaction of being able to help other people. Quite a number have heard about my recovery and have come to me for information and advice.

Some people I've spoken to have been impressed by the nutritional program but have been unable to believe that the doctors who've put them on chemotherapy could be wrong. Most of them have since died, and this saddens me because I feel their deaths were unnecessary. I only wish I'd heard about Dr. Kelley earlier and hadn't submitted myself to surgery and chemotherapy. But this, perhaps, is negative thinking. I feel grateful that I've been given the chance to get well. I feel lucky to be alive."

Dr. Kelley: **"Rosswitha brought to my attention one of the things I just take for granted and should be a characteristic of all doctors — people who're really doctors. She said, 'At last I was speaking with a doctor who treated me like an intelligent human being and was quite willing to discuss all the details of my illness.' That seems to me to be the way it should be, but I must confess at this point that I'm the one who benefits — a thousand times more than the patient does. Every single patient I've had the privilege of working with and talking to has taught me more than I could ever teach them. Patients have given to me more than I could ever give to them. The lessons I've learned working with each one have been such a beautiful experience that I just can't go on and leave it unmentioned here.**

"I find it really sad if the clinician can't learn from each patient. I can't comprehend the clinician having this phenomenal educational institution right in front of him and not learning a great deal. Not only did I learn a lot, but the people paid me to learn and I always felt a little guilty about that. I learned so much that it often seemed that I ought to be paying them. But I wouldn't have been able to function if they hadn't been paying me to be learning to do a better job each day. I certainly appreciated it and I hope it's been a feeling of mutual gain on both of our parts.

"Rosswitha brings to mind a comparison of cancer with diabetes. Before Dr. Banting and Best discovered insulin in 1918 in Canada, a person would have diabetes and would ask the doctor if it could be anything he was eating, and should he

change his diet in any way? And the doctor would say, 'Oh no, it doesn't make any difference — eat anything you want, you aren't going to live much longer anyhow, so just live it up and eat whatever you want.' Doctors couldn't connect the diet and diabetes. Even lay people in those days figured out that if you ate a lot of leafy green vegetables and reduced the amount of sugar that you took in, you survived better and did well — better than the person who didn't watch his diet.

"And so it was that after the development of insulin, doctors figured out that there's a factor in diet. In the early 1920s there weren't very good analytical facilities available. But the doctors empirically found that the people who ate green leafy vegetables and a few other foods survived diabetes much better and the sugar count in their urine was much better. They had a saying in the medical community at that time that leafy, green vegetables had 'natural insulin' in them. It wasn't actually the truth, but they became aware of the fact that including these vegetables in the diet did play a role and they were trying to explain it. We're in the same situation now with cancer. Some day in the near future, it'll dawn on the medical community that diet makes quite a difference in people with cancer and greatly affects health in general. It can't happen too soon. When it does, a lot of lives will be lived more healthfully and a lot of lives will be saved."

Breast Cancer

Violet J., Stanley, IA

7-Year Victory over Breast Cancer

"I'm a farmer's wife, age 53. We live in a modern, ranch-style home in Northeast Iowa. We raise cattle and have about 500 acres in diversified farming. We've always been active in church, farm bureau, school, and community affairs. We have four married children.

I've worked outdoors doing fieldwork, chores, chickens to tend, and a large vegetable and fruit garden. My children had lots of sickness from tonsillitis to chronic bronchitis, and coughing day and night with high fevers. When we learned about chiropractic, that helped us a lot. When our youngest daughter was 14, she missed 6 weeks of school with headaches as a forerunner of arthritis. She was in 3 different hospitals, with all the typical medical tests done, showing nothing but arthritis. They sent us home with the comment that there was nothing they could do for her arthritis but give her 6 to 20 aspirin a day. I studied nutrition like mad, gave her various things for her condition and she improved dramatically. The next year she needed a health examination so she could be a lifeguard and the doctor told us he'd never seen anyone so healthy. I told him it was all the nutrition I was giving her and he said that had nothing to do with it, but I knew it was the answer. We've had numerous medical doctors but none knew anything about nutrition or will admit it has anything to do with health.

I spent 9 years working with the American Cancer Society as door-knocker, county chairman, crusade chairman at district meetings and state conventions. My mother died of cancer. I know what the word 'cancer' means— the hopeless feeling, the despair—and I'm scared to death of it. When I made my last call on a dear friend who died of cancer, I wanted to say to her: 'I'll be the next one,' for I'd found a lump in my breast at that time; also, I was having digestive disturbances. This was three years after I started learning about nutrition. I'd read a lot of books and health magazines and I knew what medical science was doing. I was determined not to be butchered at the hospital. I said nothing to anyone about the lump; it got larger as time went on. I was trying to eat right, and to continue to gather information from books.

The following March my husband wanted to get each of us a life insurance policy. I said nothing, but knew I wouldn't pass a health test. The doctor told my husband about the lump and I was refused the insurance policy. He told me to go to the hospital and have a biopsy, but I wouldn't go. We went to visit my sister and told her. By this time the lump was plainly visible. In a few days she telephoned that she'd learned of a chiropractor who could help. He'd helped his daughter. A light in the tunnel. We started going to the chiropractor 3 times a week, a 100-mile trip. After a few calls, he told us about Dr. Kelley and advised both my sister and me to go to him, as she had had surgery and they'd found cancer. In June we made our first call to Dr. Kelley. By this time the lump in my breast was 1-3/4 inches across plus numerous small ones and even some in the other breast. I still had digestive disturbances.

Looking back now, I can see the Lord leading me to study about nutrition so I'd be prepared to know what I needed when Dr. Kelley set up our nutritional plan. I told our children of the lump in my breast and our plans to go to Texas to see Dr. Kelley. From the beginning, I had the assurance that I was doing the right thing. I'd accepted Christ as my Saviour and I knew His perfect peace and was assured of His leading. Our youngest daughter made it plain she thought I should go to a medical doctor. My husband was doubtful, but let me do what I wanted to do.

I ordered Dr. Kelley's book, **One Answer to Cancer,** *and started the beginning of the treatment, which looked like a large undertaking. Dr. Kelley was a long way off and would be hard to contact regarding problems from day to day. Still I never doubted that this was the way I should go. I'd doctored my children for 18 years with medical doctors and medicines and never had any help. This had to be the better way. I never told my family doctor about the lump in my breast; the only one who knew of it was the doctor who'd refused me the insurance policy.*

When we went to Dr. Kelley for our tests, he counseled us as long as we had questions. We left his office with our programs to follow. My sister and I studied our books all the way home, a 3-day trip. Dr. Kelley had told us in his book what to expect, how we'd feel and what our body reactions would be, so we'd be prepared for what was happening. Whenever we had doubts, we kept remembering that Dr. Kelley knew what to do.

I bought a juicer and made carrot and celery juice several times a day; that took a lot of time. Preparing all of the fresh vegetables takes time. But, I'd had my own garden for years, so I knew how much work it was to raise and prepare vegetables for the table. Now we were eating everything raw possible. Even my family cooperated.

Within two weeks, my digestive disturbances were better. At first I'd go out and work a while and come in to fix carrot juice and lay down to rest, then get up and go out again to finish the jobs. My family helped carry the water and feed for the chickens, but I still raised and dressed 150 chickens that first summer. In six weeks I felt really good, didn't have any of the things that Dr. Kelley had written in the book that I might have. My body responded quickly and I began to regain strength I hadn't had for months. **I Never Ate One Thing** *I was not supposed to eat and I took my nutrition exactly as he told me. I've always been a determined person. I did everything as near right as I could or knew to do; this helped me in my diet. If I'd even once eaten sweets or anything that was on the list of "no-no's," I* *wouldn't have been able to win the game. That's what you need — determination to follow the rules.*

In six months the lumps in my breasts were gone. I felt much better than I had before. I'd not had surgery and the awful ordeal of that, or intravenous feeding, and I still had a whole body. I was telling everyone to eat right. But I did not tell anyone (outside of my family) that I had cancer. People knew I'd been really sick, but not what was really wrong with me. I guess I wanted to be sure myself that I could do it before I'd tell anyone you could lick cancer with proper lifestyle and nutrition. I continued chiropractic treatment for years, and still do. Mostly when I talk to people about eating properly — not eating food with preservatives, eating raw foods instead of cooked ones — they make light of it and never really listen. Yet, many call me with all of their ills and ask me what they should do. Some I can advise and some don't believe what you say, anyway.

Three years later in March I applied to an agent for another insurance policy with another company. I told him I'd been refused a policy because of the lumps in my breast. He sent me for another health examination with another doctor. I told this doctor about the lumps — that I did not go to a doctor, but started taking nutrition and eating raw foods, etc. and the lumps went away. He couldn't find any lumps. They X-rayed my chest and found nothing. Yet he wouldn't believe the nutrition had anything to do with it. He told me I was in excellent health and I got the insurance policy. It was a much larger policy than the one I'd been refused because of the lumps in my breast.

In July after the X-rays, I again noticed the lumps in my breast. I had just read an article in the paper that they were finding "hard evidence that X-rays are actually causing cancer." On July 20, 1976, when I discovered the lumps back again, I immediately went back on my original schedule and diet and within 6 months my lumps were again gone. My advice to others would be — Don't get X-rays taken. The radiation exposure is too dangerous.

After 5 years with Dr. Kelley I don't need tests as often as I did. I follow his diet list and my own home-grown foods when possible. I continue to take all kinds of nutrition, as he recommends. I'm not as strict with my diet as I was the first three years but when I don't eat right or stop the nutrition, I don't feel good and I know what to do to get better again. Dr. Kelley's answered personally all my letters to him about health problems that come up. He takes my telephone calls when I need to know something right away. Good health is something you need to work at daily. Dr. Kelley's advice works. My illness has given my husband and me a better, closer relationship than we've ever known. I know Metabolic Medicine works; it did for me."

Dr. Kelley: **"It's hard to appreciate the sorts of obstacles patients had to overcome to see me as a clinician. First of all, I'm not a medical doctor. I'm a dentist. Second, my office was unbelievably unacceptable when compared to where a lot of these people had gone — to the great clinics and hospitals of our world. They really had to lower themselves to come into my meager surroundings. While adequately appointed and kept immaculately clean by my receptionist, there certainly was no pretension. On many occasions people would drive up in their Cadillacs or Rolls Royces and drive away because they thought that they couldn't possibly find anything of worth in such an unpretentious office."**

Pancreatic Cancer

Donnella Z., Amarillo, TX

8-Year Victory over Pancreatic Cancer

The parents of the patient relate the following testimony:

"**Our daughter is age 27 with no history of smoking, drinking or drugs. She had an attack of hypoglycemia between ages of 15-17.**

November 1973 (when D was 20) was our first indication of a problem. She was stricken with aches, pains and fever. A 3-day flu had been hitting our area with similar symptoms so at this point, we weren't overly concerned. After several days of unsuccessfully trying to keep her temperature down, we decided this was something other than the flu. At the emergency receiving room of our hospital, chest X-rays, blood tests and urinalysis failed to locate her problem. Her temperature range for a 24-hour period went from below normal to 106°F. We were referred to a M.D. who specialized in internal medicine.

Thus began a nightmare that lasted many weeks. Testing for one week as an outpatient ended in no answers. She was rapidly going downhill — weakened by the many hospital trips. We were advised to admit her for extensive testing. Up to this point in our lives we'd never even considered the fact that anyone could be this sick and not have a physician give the reason. We feared in the beginning a serious disease, but as time went on, would've welcomed a concrete answer. Watching D dying for no apparent reason left us quite helpless except for our faith in God. As time went on, we found ourselves doing more praying to God and less reaching out to Man for answers. We needed a miracle and had no doubt where that would come from.

Biopsies, scans, X-rays, bone marrow tests and blood taken every two hours became our way of life for the next 10 days. No answers. D was losing ground. Six local doctors and two consulting doctors from a larger city failed to find anything that could be causing her illness. By now D had lost 40 pounds, most of her hair had fallen out, her menstrual periods had stopped, severe anemia and painful hot lumps traveled all over her body. Massive doses of penicillin and streptomycin had caused a near-total hearing loss. She was dying from malnutrition.

The week before Christmas the doctor informed us that D had run out of time. The only thing left was exploratory surgery. After questioning the doctor closely about her chances of coming through the surgery and of their chances in finding the problem, we decided to take her home, a big decision. If she was going to die, we wanted her to be at home where her loved ones could be with her. No more tests and definitely no hospital. We left for home with a lung fungus medication although all tests were negative.

Little did we know that this would be the turning point in our battle. Everything was downhill from there out except for one minor incident. We were on our own now but somehow had a strange feeling of relief. We had no intention of just sitting and waiting; we couldn't just do nothing. We began with Adelle Davis' anti-stress formula and large dosages of vitamin C — (the hospital doctor had refused to give D any vitamin C injection while in the hospital.) We'd been taking natural vitamins for several years and knew vitamin C would do no harm. As we look back, we know that this was God's way of letting us know we were finally on the right track. Many people all over the USA were praying which resulted in two tired weary people getting divine guidance directly from God daily.

Five days after the vitamin C was given, her temperature was normal. God in His simplicity, restored life to a dying body.

Our first visit to the doctor's office three weeks later found D improved in every area: Strong enough to walk, hair growing, appetite normal and gaining weight. The doctor's face could not hide his disbelief. His associates came for a look-see too. After we explained what we'd done, he checked her records and gave all the credit to the fungus medication. He was so sure and convincing, we made our first blunder since leaving their hospital. We cut back on the vitamin C and concentrated on the medication. Her temperature rose immediately. We were shook. After asking God's forgiveness, we resumed with our vitamin C schedule, adding health-building foods as fast as D could take them.

A searching time began as we looked for answers. D was returning to health as rapidly as she went down, but what happened? Would it happen again? Did God want us to go on searching for the answer or accept her healing and let it go at that? God led our steps to the answer. Because we were involved in a natural business, we had heard of Dr. Kelley. Thinking he could help us with a proper balanced diet that would be scientific instead of guesswork, we began to investigate the possibility of a visit. We'd exhausted our finances paying hospital and doctor fees, so it was back to earnest praying. When we received a check from a friend in the amount that we needed for the trip, we knew God had given us a green light.

In March our first visit to Dr. Kelley was made. We couldn't believe what took place. Answers instead of questions. How refreshing! There was a problem: A malignant tumor on her pancreas; it was still there. Wasn't God good to keep us searching? (A medical doctor later confirmed the tumor.) Although saddened by the nature of her problem, we were relieved to finally have an answer. We were told when her problem started, how long it'd take to clear it and a possible reason for the problem beginning in the first place. The diet alone would've been worth the trip; the rest we considered priceless.

Upon our return we began to change our lifestyle to fit D's new program. It was difficult, but we followed it in its entirety without any alterations. D had amazingly few problems and returned to work June 1. (A total leave-of-absence of 6 months.) To date she's had no recurrence of cancer and no major health problems of any nature. She takes vitamin and mineral supplements.

What we've learned about cancer through Dr. Kelley has spared at least 8 lives. We'd go the same route again well knowing what we'd be getting into and knowing the results. D's life was worth it all; the other 8 we look at as a major bonus from the Lord. My unanswered question: Why could Dr. Kelley find in one day what many doctors couldn't find in many months?"

Dr. Kelley: **"Pancreatic cancer is devastating and close to my heart because that's what I had. The average life expectancy of a clinically diagnosed case of pancreas malignancy is 2 months. This lovely young lady, with 8 years' survival, is an example of what can be done with total family unity. This family is a wonderful example of 'how to.' They addressed two contributing factors to successful healing—a positive attitude and the willingness to do whatever it takes to get well.**

Pancreatic cancer has some particular characteristics which are not like other cancers. These characteristics include a lot of excessive gas and unusual mental

states such as severe nightmares, depression, anxiety and all the negative factors that otherwise happy and cheerful individuals wouldn't have. Such individuals flip into depression and irritation and become hard to get along with.

"D's so nice, it's hard to imagine her being hard to get along with. But even if she was, her parents would've understood and paid no attention. That kind of unselfish support can make the difference between life and death."

Skin Cancer

Betty F., Spokane, WA

11-Year Victory over Skin Cancer

You have cancer.

"When I heard those three words over the telephone, my only thought was, 'I'm going to die!' I was so 'shook up,' I barely heard the voice on the other end of the telephone tell me to come in and see Dr. S.L. as soon as possible. Only another cancer patient knows what it means to be told, 'you have cancer.' It's not only a sentence of death; it's a sentence of death linked with severe pain.

I was 46, living and working in New York City when I was diagnosed as having cancer. I'd been feeling "poorly" since I was 37 and had had a partial hysterectomy. I was trying every day to live with "feeling poorly," because no doctor I saw was able to help me "feel better." And believe me, I saw many physicians in the "Big Apple."

Our family physician, Dr. H.H., said I should see a specialist because my periods were too long, I was losing too much blood during each period and had fibroids. I went to the specialist he recommended, who urged me not to wait, but to have the operation "before it was too late." I followed order and I had the operation. (By the way, I remember being sedated and prepared in the morning for the operation, which was scheduled for 1:00 p.m. I remember not being wheeled in until 4:00 p.m.! I was worried and wondered . . . will I get the right operation? This experience filled me with dismay and created distrust for the medical profession.)

I was discharged with a clean bill of health. Now that I'd had the operation, did I feel better? No, I felt worse! I was passing gas, feeling tired and terribly constipated. It did no good to hear nice words of assurance from the doctor or that the tumor they'd removed was the size of a 5-month pregnancy. I didn't feel better hearing that it was normal for some people not to have daily bowel movements. I felt loggy. Shortly after the operation and an "OK checkup" from the surgeon, I went to our family physician with the complaint, "I have pain in the abdomen." He examined me and was surprised to find a cyst in the former womb area. He asked me to return to the specialist but I refused, I telling our family physician that my confidence in the specialist was gone. I asked him to take care of me. After much pleading, he did. He removed the cyst in his office by cauterization. Those were two painful office visits for me.

I still felt rotten, fatigued all the time and passing gas much of the time. I had attacks of illness diagnosed as myositis and facial neuritis. I had pains in my abdomen, which were diagnosed as a nervous stomach. The family doctor suggested I take the gallbladder test. Fortunately, at the time, there was nothing wrong with my gallbladder. I went to the dentist often, because my gums were bleeding and my teeth were loose.

I was born with a brown mole on my left cheek. When I was 14, hair began to grow in the mole. It didn't hurt, but I felt a pulsating sensation in the mole area. I saw a doctor who recommended removing the hairs by electrolysis. Afterward, the doctor said, "It looks OK; we'll leave it alone for now, but you should always watch the mole for any changes."

Two years after the hysterectomy operation at the age of 39, the brown mole on my left check started to throb and grow. I saw a skin specialist and had the mole excised. A biopsy was performed: Diagnosis: Non-malignant.

In the fall of 1969 I saw a gynecologist for a checkup. This doctor recommended estrogen because I had had a partial hysterectomy. I took the estrogen for 3 months only because round white spots emerged on both of my thighs and a growth developed under the arch of my left foot which I had to have surgically removed. This, too, was biopsied and declared non-malignant. At the same time the skin specialist removed some small growths on my face, forehead and right wrist.

I was depressed: I was still suffering with passing gas; my eyes were deteriorating and couldn't focus; couldn't see telephone numbers or addresses in the telephone book; found it difficult to read the newspapers; suffered with muscle weakness and cramps. The latter condition would often strike at night while I was sleeping with such severity that I'd wake up screaming from the pain. My chestnut-brown hair was turning gray; the texture was now brittle. Worst of all, my face "itched" 24 hours a day. I wanted to holler, because there was no letup of pain. I found I could no longer tolerate any sunlight.

I went to yet another specialist and I gave him a list of my complaints. He gave me a battery of tests, a big bill, and said that the tests showed there was nothing wrong with me. He said, "You're getting older. Try to take things easier." He suggested I see a psychiatrist. I questioned him about my facial condition. He said the facial problem was probably part of my active imagination. Ooh, but I was angry when I left his office.

I found the pain in my face intolerable made an appointment with a skin specialist in 1971. He performed surgery in his office and said, 'We'll do a biopsy but I doubt that you'll get your money's worth,' Well, his office is the party that called and told me, 'You have cancer.' I was shocked sure that I had a charmed existence when it came to surgery and biopsies. After all, I'd been through many operations and biopsies and all had been diagnosed as being benign. I followed the skin specialist's recommendation of going into the hospital immediately and having the "entire cancerous tumor completely removed." He said he was sure this would be the case.

The short hospital stay was an ordeal. For a facial condition I had to undergo a series of body X-rays and other tests. When I asked, the reason, I was told it was 'hospital procedure.' I don't know what good they did; I do know it hiked the bill. In the hospital I had a section between my lip and chin cut again. This biopsy also stated that 'the patient has cancer.' The doctor said, 'Go home. Let your face heal and see me in six months.'

About this time I began to visit health food stores in my neighborhood. Why? I thought there might be something to taking supplements. I was hoping to find something to take to have more energy. I bought books on health and health magazines. I was investigating another avenue towards feeling better.

I didn't wait six months to see the doctor. I called for an appointment 4 months later because of the continuing pain. I saw the skin specialist and on January 14, 1972, he cut away another portion of my chin. Another biopsy was performed. Diagnosis: Cancer. He now told me that I should see another type of specialist. In his opinion, I now needed chemo-surgery, because the cancer had metastasized and evidently was deeper than he had previously thought. He explained the treatment to me. I would be under the care of a well-known chemotherapy specialist. I'd not have to be hospitalized for the treatment, but go to the hospital for 5 to 10 days on a daily basis from 9:00 a.m. to 5:00 p.m. Special chemicals would be put on my face and where an area revealed cancer, the specialist would cut. After following this procedure, he told me that if my face didn't heal he knew of a good plastic surgeon.

For several reasons I decided not to follow the above path. First, the expense was beyond the means of my husband and myself, and second, female vanity. I couldn't bear to think of going out shopping, or to work with a face any more mutilated with scars and blobs than I already had from previous facial operations described above. I must mention here that after the second facial surgery, when the bandages were removed, instead of a scar there was a big blue eruption on my skin, which I named, "The Blue Blob." The surgeon said it was the 'cancer showing.' I reasoned that since neither the surgeon nor the skin specialist had cured me — even though I was assured of a cure with each bit of surgery I went through — I was fearful of following the road many of my relatives had. Too many in my family have died of cancer. I can remember hearing the doctors assure them and members of the family that they'd recover. Doctors assure cancer patients they'll recover till the day the cancer patients die.

The surgeon/skin specialist recommending chemo-surgery wanted me to start treatment immediately. I had quite a time telling him I couldn't do this immediately, that I had to take care of business and personal matters first. It was difficult, but I finally convinced him it wasn't necessary for me to quickly hop into the chemo-surgery program. I promised to call him soon and let him know when I'd start the chemo-surgery program. I never did call him, but his nurse and even he called my husband, urging him to reason with me 'for my own good.'

Right after receiving the 'black news,' I called my husband at work and told him I wouldn't be back at our place of business or home until I found another way to combat cancer. Don't laugh at me. I knew there must be a way to fight cancer without being cut, burned or poisoned any more. In the summer of 1971 my husband was tutoring in Connecticut. While he was out working one sunny afternoon and I was alone in our hotel room, for the first time in my life I prayed to God for help. I cried and prayed at the same time. I cried because I was in so much pain. I let it all out because I was alone and no one could hear me. I prayed out loud, prayed silently. I kept repeating, "If there's a God, then help me find the person who can help me get well." I fell asleep crying and when I woke, I thought, "Soon I'll find a way to fight cancer.

While I was talking to my husband, it came to me that my prayers for help would be answered by visiting a health store in my neighborhood that carried a varied selection of books on the subject of health, including cancer. Also, this health store posted notices of health meetings which I noted from time to time, but never attended because I was working when the meetings were held.

After talking with my husband, I took a subway to the health store and read the first four pages of the Kelley book, One Answer to Cancer, and became very excited because the symptoms Dr. Kelley described in a cancer patient matched mine except for the hernia. That condition I didn't have. I begged and pleaded with the owner of the health store to help me get to Dr. Kelley. She listened but did not answer. I told her I was sure she knew how to help me get the Kelley Test. I broke down and cried and told her I had cancer. Then she gave me the name of a person to contact.

I had my first Kelley Test in late January of 1972. The Kelley Test disclosed that I had only one tumor in the jaw area of my face. Imagine, dear reader, Dr. Kelley told me the location of my cancer sight unseen. He told me the location without subjecting me to painful surgery or biopsies. I say shame on the medical profession for ignoring Dr. Kelley.

The first day I began the Kelley regime I took the Epsom salt 'cocktail' and collapsed on my kitchen floor. Yes, I was that full of garbage; I know that today. All my life, until I started the Kelley program, I hadn't eaten food to nourish my body, only American junk food — French fries, pizza, soft drinks, potato chips.

The Kelley program's not at all similar to any program devised today by the medical Establishment. You don't take a pill or a few pills; you don't get a shot or a few shots. By golly, you have to WORK to get well. I experienced many unpleasant, unusual conditions I've never experienced before. I had migraine headaches, and all too often, because I went overly 'gung-ho' on the program. I developed 'flu-like body aches.' The Kelley program of purges, enemas and colonics, cleaning the liver, kidneys and lungs, changing one's diet — shook up my body — literally. At times I could feel my insides turn upside down. Often I felt so 'goopy' ill I'd complain, "Ooh, how can Dr. Kelley do this to me?" when really what I was saying was, 'Ooh, how did I ever get this sick? I eliminated parasites and even live worms. Our apartment acquired a putrid odor. But then I started having days without passing gas. And days when I felt as young as a 12-year-old. Then I'd have some rotten, rotten days of feeling just plain punky.

I started the Kelley program set up for me in February of 1972 I think it's important to note that the cancer I had changed from cancer to a sebaceous cyst and then to a mydiox or mucus cyst. When my body was ready, according to the Kelley Test, I had the mydiox cyst cut out by yet another surgeon, Dr. W. in 1974 — "The Blue Blob" which one Dr. told me I'd have to learn to live with was removed. And, yes, my face was no longer a mass of scars.

The family physician, Dr. H.H., who was preparing my husband to accept my coming demise, just couldn't believe the change in my face. When he saw the cancer was no longer there, he said, 'My diagnosis and the biopsies were wrong; we were all mistaken. You never had cancer.' I just couldn't believe his attitude: I can only guess that because of his medical training, he couldn't see beyond "The Establishment.' It's also my guess that if he were to recognize a non-toxic therapy, it'd negate his schooling and work and further, it'd be mentally painful because he's lost many patients from the dreaded disease of cancer.

Three years ago, in 1975 my husband and I left New York City and now reside in Spokane, Washington. We left the tall canyons of the buildings in New York City for the tall evergreens of Washington State.

I'm lucky; I no longer have to combat the pollution that exists in New York City. I find living in a smaller city compatible with my health. I enjoy the beauty of nature — birds nesting in an evergreen in our backyard, cats meowing, dogs barking, crickets chirping. It's lots better music to my ears and soul than the honking of cabs and cars, the sirens of police and fire trucks.

I work full-time. Clean my own house, do the laundry, cooking and gardening. I enjoy my grandchildren and am happy to be alive. I'm grateful and say thanks in my prayers every day for Dr. and Mrs. William Donald Kelley and the Kelley Program."

Dr. Kelley: **"Betty brings to mind one of the important features of the current cancer situation: Many people prefer to do nothing than to go through being tortured by chemotherapy and radiation and mutilated by surgery. They just ask for pain medication and leave. Interestingly, studies have proven that you last longer if you do nothing, rather than take a lot of the treatments that go on at this time.**

"We're coming to a time, particularly in our country, where there's hardly a family that hasn't lost a close friend or relative to cancer. And the family has watched this person go from fairly robust good health to a skeleton and be tortured by the treatments. When you've had one or two friends or relatives go that way and the doctor tells you that you have cancer, you don't jump right into the next operating room or in front of the next X-ray machine that rolls by. You think about it, you consider it, you remember your friends' or relatives' stories and give it a lot of serious thought."

Bone Cancer

Ina S., West, FL

9-Year Victory over Bone Cancer

"I'd like to tell others what Dr. Kelley's book, One Answer to Cancer, did for a number of us, but more especially just how it began with me.

Doctors had tenderly, but emphatically, told me that they could do nothing for my condition. It was apparently cancer of the bone — and as lovingly as a father, with tears in his eyes, one doctor said: 'You'll get worse until — ?' He left me immediately. Somehow I didn't feel shaken at all. I felt so secure in God's hands. I knew the doctor in the clinic had told my son that it was a matter of 3 to 6 months that the spine was hopelessly deteriorating and nine vertebrae were collapsed, causing cramps across my shoulders and chest. When the attacks came, I was in such pain and had to have pain-killing relief. And had these tablets had such severe side effects that I could scarcely endure them.

My bones were brittle and, as the doctors told my son, were like chalk. So small a pressure as a bump of my elbow against my ribs would crack a rib. Faith in God as my greatest physician helped me to hold steady, until one day I was touched by His healing power. The healing was instantaneous as to the pain and spine. Doctors couldn't believe this but I never took an aspirin or any narcotic. There was no pain or cramps. The spine was healed.

At this time Dr. Kelley's book, One Answer to Cancer, was laid on a table near my bed. I picked it up two or three times. Finally, I realized I was not gaining strength but the opposite was true. However, I never had another pain in my spine or cramps. So I read from Dr. Kelley's book these words: 'Malignancy indicates an active pancreatic enzyme deficiency.' I began in earnest to read. Every word sounded so logical and clear. Cancer always seemed like a killer that couldn't be controlled. The killer was too complex. But Dr. Kelley had the key. He was unselfish and tried to put the key on the lowest shelf where all of us, little or big, intelligent or uninformed could reach the key to one answer! The diet and nutritional program cost a bit, but nothing compared to the fruitless efforts of the medical doctors and hospitals. So, on my bed of affliction, growing weaker all the way, I set myself to follow each step of Dr. Kelley's instructions.

Many times I thought, 'Perhaps I am wrong in following Dr. Kelley's diet and nutritional program.' Our medical doctors wouldn't listen when I told them about it. But, feeling I had nothing to lose, I kept on. Dr. Kelley's book is most valuable. Here, I who knew nothing, was free from those painful unprof-

itable visits to the doctor's office. Eating differently was never a problem for me — I had been a missionary for 40 years. If a diet would help, I thought I should get on it as strictly as Dr. Kelley suggested — and not just keep eating anything I felt like eating. So I took everything seriously. One year later I felt much better, was up and out on the road in the missionary services, traveling 20,000 miles one summer. However, I felt the need of some guidance, so I went to see Dr. Kelley. It had been a constant battle to keep on a strict and proper diet with the stress and strain of my work.

I've gone abroad three times and carried a heavy workload in the U.S.A. to visit among hundreds abroad and at home, and to not eat 'junk' food takes a backbone of steel and a conviction that this nutritional program is best. Stress and strain go with the public appearances and directional work but these five years have been good years, although they were not without battles. But I'm able to work 12 hours nearly every day but Sunday.

Even if members of our family and missionary group have no cancer, my husband and I urge all to consider the value of a nutritional diet as a way of life and health. Our grandchildren are being taught the importance of proper diets, purges and careful living. There are those around us who are dying of cancer unnecessarily. We've suggested the Kelley Nutritional Program to people we've seen in need, but many have refused to put that much effort into regaining their health and are now gone. We've seen others who've willingly read Dr. Kelley's book in time, found the key and are living examples today of what his program can do."

Dr. Kelley: **"When the doctor says you have cancer, he gets your attention rather rapidly and God gets our attention rather rapidly. We address God immediately. Then we realize God's been talking to us all along, we just haven't been listening. He's been trying to communicate with us in several ways short of violating our own free will. The reason that He created us is to let us experience life, to have free will and to come to Him voluntarily and with love and appreciation — not by force, but because of the love that is in our hearts.**

As we address the situation of cancer, we realize that we did it to ourselves and this is, to me, the chief characteristic of God — His respect for our free will. It's one of the greatest lessons I've learned through the cancer situation, through my cancer. God in all of His wisdom and comprehension and completeness and knowingness doesn't force us to do anything — to be right, to do right to be kind to each other — to do anything. He's set the rules, the requirements, and the example of how we should conduct our life activities, but we're so dumb we can't figure it all out. He's given us great freedom. He has respect for our beings and our persons. He allows us the privilege of getting into trouble. When we do get into trouble we turn around and blame God. Those of us who get into trouble with cancer are learning a pretty tough lesson, but we get the message eventually. When we get the message that it's our fault, we turn, and in our pride and haughtiness and all the other things that go along with the proper description of us, we humble ourselves and vow ourselves to reality and truth and righteousness, and then God can talk to us. I just hope those who learn this lesson, as most of my counselees have, don't have to learn it again. Or suffer some other tragedy."

Prostate and Rectal Cancer

Walter M., Daytona Beach, FL

11-Year Victory over Prostate and Rectal Cancer

"When I fully realized that the forthcoming biopsy would reveal a malignancy, my emotions completely overwhelmed me. That horrible thought which had plagued me for years could and would come true.

For many years prior to the actual operation, I'd been bothered with prostatitis. But with the absence of information and having a strong, youthful body, any thought of potential problems was quickly dismissed. These were things that always happened to the "other guy. As the years passed, the problem became more acute and visits to the urologist became more frequent. My attitude then changed to one of concern.

I was granted a brief respite from worry after a needle biopsy showed there was no malignancy. But still, there was the burning and discomfort that intensified when my wife and I would take long trips by car. The embarrassment of having to urinate regardless of passing traffic played havoc with my nerves. There was a time when it became so irritating it was necessary to visit a clinic in another state while traveling in order to obtain relief. And it was the usual prescription of antibiotics. But it did provide temporary relief.

One night while preparing to retire, I sat on the edge of the bed to remove my shoes. A pain in the rectal area surpassed all other pain. It was impossible to sit. After an emergency visit to our family physician brought relief, I returned to the urologist and was told there was a nodule on the prostate. This news didn't cause me any great concern until I read about the possibility of cancer when a nodule appears. My procrastination forced my wife to make an appointment for me with a local urologist. My medical records were sent to him and after an examination and consultation, he informed me that I needed surgery.

After the operation and a painful recuperative period my self-confidence was beginning to resurface. But the following year a devastating bombshell exploded. There was a definite recurrence, which manifested itself in the rectal area. When the second operation was over and my period of recuperation felt complete, another horrible and terrifying jolt came an elevation in the acid-phosphatase reading. It was then I felt totally defeated and resigned to my fate as another victim of cancer. However, this resignation was not gracefully accepted. My emotions gave way and negative thinking controlled me.

Our son contacted a health food storeowner who, by the Grace of God, was familiar with the Kelley Program. After much insistence by my family, my wife and I visited Dr. Kelley. The first visit in 1974 was overwhelming when I saw the amount of vitamins that were necessary for return to good health. There were anxious moments of nausea, dizziness and apprehension regarding its effectiveness. But it has proven to be the most significant step I ever made. Since that first visit all medical tests and X-rays have been negative.

Each day I pray silently and openly, to thank God, our Creator, for His divine guidance in leading me to Dr. Kelley. God does act in mysterious ways, and when obeying His natural laws, we all prosper. And today at age 67, my life's more complete than ever, God, in his loving ways, has granted me the ability to enjoy His great outdoors. Above all, my spiritual life has risen to greater heights in my love and appreciation of Him."

Dr. Kelley: **"Walter brings to mind that cancer, or any degenerative condition, doesn't all of a sudden happen: it takes a long time to get there. You get sicker and sicker and it isn't all of a sudden you wake up one morning with a full-blown cancer. Instead, you've gradually earned every bit of it by your lifestyle or by the dumb things you've done, and the abuse you put your body through. We earn cancer just as we make either A's or F's on our report cards. Walter also reminds me that in our society we do tell the patient that he has cancer, which I think is a much better attitude than in the European society where they do not tell the patient. You go to a doctor and he'll never tell you what's wrong with you. He'll let you die and then tell your relatives after you're dead that you had cancer. If you were never told, what choice did you have?**

The word 'choice' brings to mind our former Vice-President, Hubert Humphrey, who was a cancer victim. I talked to a close friend of Senator Humphrey who said that when Humphrey had a chance to carry out non-toxic therapy, he wanted very much to do so. But he couldn't because he thought he'd set a bad example by not supporting our medical monopoly. He wouldn't be supporting the National Cancer Institute, the National Cancer Society and the AMA. He was essentially a sacrificial lamb — as is everybody who goes through the torture and inquisitions. He knew he had a choice and chose not to exercise a preferred alternative — a real tragedy."

Colon and Liver Cancer

Mabel H., Longview, WA

8-Year Victory over Colon and Liver Cancer

"Health is something I'd enjoyed for many years, something I'd taken for granted, and something I hadn't cherished as I ought. During the fall of 1974, I experienced a tired feeling at the end of my day's work and often found it necessary to rest before preparing my evening meal. At the beginning of February I had a complete physical and Dr. X gave this verdict, "You have a clean slate of health." I shook my head and he asked me why. I proceeded to explain this distressed feeling in my lower abdomen. The barium enema, which followed, revealed the cancer in the colon. You can imagine what thoughts arose within me but I'm thankful I've learned, in a measure, to accept disappointments, too. Our pathway's not always going to be sunny and bright.

After the colostomy, the surgeon discovered I had cancer of the liver, which was inoperable. He recommended I have chemotherapy and an appointment was made to see the oncologist. In the mean-time, my daughter, who lives in Iowa, contacted a few people who had cancer and had received great help using the Kelley Nutritional Plan. She called me and asked what I wanted to do; that wasn't a hard decision since I'd been aware of this type of cancer treatment. Nevertheless Mary and I went to talk to Dr. W. (the oncologist). He was a real gentleman and didn't put forth a successful picture of chemotherapy. He wished me the best and said he'd never heard of the Kelley Nutritional Plan. My daughter also had to call the surgeon to tell him my decision. He made it clear that this was not in accordance with the American Medical Association procedure, and this, of course, we understood. Am I ever thankful to my daughter that she got in contact with people who'd proved that Dr. Kelley's Plan really did work in bringing people back to health!

My daughter helped me in filling out Dr. Kelley's questionnaire. There was a question or two I couldn't answer, so she called Dr. X to ask. His manner of speech was shocking. The language he used was such no doctor would need to use to answer a question or two concerning my physical checkup. His attitude toward my decision was distasteful. Dr. X is my doctor no more!

About seven weeks after my surgery, I made my first visit to Dr. Kelley at the end of March. The night before my appointment with him I got the flu so you can imagine in what shape I was. My Kelley Index was 720 and my body was so deficient in every respect. I felt very comfortable in Dr. Kelley's presence, but having my daughter with me gave me courage.

Before I reached home I had a distiller, juicer and the necessary vitamins and supplements. Then started my new way of living. To a degree I understood the discomfort I could experience because I'd read Dr. Kelley's book. I made a tremendous change from my former way of preparing my food. I became quite time-conscious, since I needed some supplements every 2 hours during the day and in the middle of the night when my alarm helped me out. I had a great number of supplements plus all the carrot juice, seeds, nuts, boiled eggs, yogurt, etc. I'd lost much weight, but quite soon began to gain. I kept on the program for at least 10 days — more if possible — and then vacationed for five days. I had much to learn in the giving of enemas. A coffee enema makes you feel clean and refreshed.

This program required much systematic work but I had a goal in view, God had spared my life during surgery and now with His help, I could face the future. Every day I asked for guidance, wisdom and courage to walk and live as I ought to so He'd be pleased with me here on earth and throughout the endless ages of eternity. My relatives and friends all encouraged me to keep on the program. There was no opposition. If you feel a course is right, you'll pursue it. This is true spiritually, too. The outside pressure isn't going to defeat you.

At the end of the 8 months I made my second visit to Dr. Kelley and this time, my Index was 420,- 300 less than my initial visit. We all jumped for joy. April 1978, my Index was 10! I'm a very thankful person.

This body God has given is a marvelous piece of creation; it functions so perfectly, isn't it only right that we should feed and care for it properly?"

Dr. Kelley: "Mabel is a friend of several years and fellow-member of our Christian fellowship. She had colon and liver cancer. The colon and liver are two of the main detoxification systems helping us get rid of toxins. Unfortunately, they themselves are high on the list of organs attacked by cancer. Metabolic Medicine is built around natural processes, of which proper health of the colon and liver and the proper detoxification of the body are major factors. Like Mabel, we all take good

health for granted and never think about having bad health until it hits us. Particularly in the case of cancer, we think: 'It'll happen to someone else. It'll never happen to me.' We try to not even imagine the prospect since it's so dreadful.

A lot of times we're like the proverbial ostrich that sticks its head in the sand. We don't want to know about it, trying to ignore it so it'll go away. However, as God's children, we owe it to ourselves and to God to take care of our bodies. It may cost a little money at first, but it'll actually save money in the long run to take time out of your life and address the cancer issue. Do the Self-Test every 9 to 12 months so that if you ever develop cancer, you'll discover it early.

Mabel's experience with Dr. W. is really more typical than her experience with Dr. X. Most family doctors, the ones out on the firing line, have our best interests at heart. Generally it's not the local family doctor that gives us problems; it's the massive, impersonal medical Establishment."

Spleen, Pancreas and Lung Cancer

Rachael S., Norcross, GA

26-Year Victory over Cancer of the Spleen, Pancreas and Left Lung.

Dr. Kelley spoke with Rachael in July, 2000. For 28 years she has told everyone she meets who has a health problem about the Kelley Program. Rachael wants everyone to know that it is because of Dr. Kelley that she has lived to love and enjoy four grandchildren and has recently become great-grandma to twins. The following is her story:

"On September 28, 1971 I was admitted to the hospital as an emergency case suffering with acute severe abdominal pain. The next morning I was taken to the operating room for an emergency exploratory with subsequent removal of an abscessed right ovary and fallopian tube (my healthy appendix was also removed). I was told I had peritonitis. Several days later after X-rays of the colon I was told I had three tumors in the hepatic flexure of the transverse colon. The doctor said he was "pretty sure at least one was malignant" and I must be scheduled for colon resection in 30 days. I asked him what could be done if further surgery proved inadequate. He said they'd give me cobalt.

On the way home and during the next few days I pondered my predicament. I was in emotional shock and weak and sick in body. Mentally, I reviewed my symptoms over the past months. My health had deteriorated gradually. For at least a year, I'd been unable to sleep on my left side and more recently, unable to sleep on my back. I felt a pressure-like discomfort in the left upper quadrant and under the left rib cage. I also experienced shortness of breath when in these positions. I had "night sweats," awakening frequently at 1:00 or 2:00 a.m. drenched in perspiration. I had a persistent backache and low energy level. In the previous six months I'd lost 40 pounds. I was 45 years of age and, as a registered nurse, had nursed hundreds of cancer patients in various stages of the disease. I recalled some painful statistics. The survival rate for metastatic cancer was less than 1%.

Later, I learned the primary tumor was in the spleen with involvement in the pancreas and lower left lung as well as metastasis to the colon. I had a difficult decision to make. I felt my body was too weak to withstand major surgery again in four weeks and yet my surgeon had told me I would be "very foolish" not to consent to further surgery. In my helplessness I claimed God's promises in James 1:5; 'If any of you lack wisdom, let him ask of God that giveth to all men liberally.' As is often the case, God had already begun to answer my prayer before I asked. Six months prior to my hospitalization, I'd read Dr. Kelley's book, One Answer To Cancer, and was so impressed I told a friend, 'If I ever have cancer, I think this is the treatment I'd follow.' Little did I realize that within 6 months, I'd be faced with that decision. My ultimate decision was to go see Dr. Kelley with the thought that I'd postpone the surgery until I could get my body built up on a good nutritional program.

I went on Dr. Kelley's program in November of 1971. My malignancy index was 700. I sent in a urine specimen to Dr. Contreras in Mexico. The test for malignancy was positive. I realized my weak body was fighting three major battles — recovering from the trauma of surgery and peritonitis, cancer, and severe emotional stress. Every 3 to 5 weeks I suffered a healing crisis, usually lasting about 5 days. During this time I stopped taking my enzymes. My symptoms were an ache-all-over feeling, nausea, abdominal pain, weakness and mental depression. I used zone therapy, hot salt baths and hot wet baths for pain control to avoid taking pill medication. My family provided great assistance and moral support. Friends and neighbors often brought fresh vegetables, fruits and nuts; some even supplied fresh, non-chlorinated water. Many prayers were uttered on my behalf.

After three months, I went back to Dr. Kelley. In spite of all the suffering since the last visit, I felt I was making progress. The test confirmed that in fact I had made remarkable progress. I decided not to have further surgery, unless some emergency situation arose such as symptoms of intestinal obstruction.

I continued to improve. My healing crises became further and further apart and less severe. My checkup every 3 months with Dr. Kelley showed remarkable progress. In September of 1972 my local physician checked my condition. My blood chemistry was normal, colon X-rays were negative and physical examinations revealed nothing abnormal. Twenty-eight months later I completed another series of tests; X-rays, Pap smear, etc.; all were completely negative. By this time my night sweats had disappeared and I could sleep comfortably in any position. I'd gained 20 pounds, and my general health and sense of well-being was better than it'd been in fifteen years.

I'm indebted to Dr. Kelley and his kind and wonderful staff and grateful to God that an alternative has been provided for cancer patients who choose not to undergo radiation, chemotherapy or surgery."

Dr. Kelley: "Rachael and her husband and I have been friends for a long time. One of the blessings that I've had over these years, along with some of the problems inherent in helping to change the course of health care in our society, is the friends and friendships that I've been permitted to have. Rachel reminds all of those who start on this program that they'll have a lot of 'up' days and many, many 'down' days. It's hard, and it's painful and it takes a lot of energy and faith to continue. There's a lot of pain involved."

Pancreas and Liver Cancer

W. D. Kelley, D.D.S., Winfield, KS

38-Year (38 in 2001) Victory over Pancreatic/Liver Cancer

I can truthfully say that I've cured or healed myself of cancer (malignancy) and I can cure myself again if it ever becomes necessary. Better still, I've learned God's Law of Health concerning malignancy (cancer) and will ever invoke this Law so that I'm not likely to have the disease again.

In the old adage, "Physician, heal thyself," two things stand out to me. One is, if a physician can't heal himself, how can he heal others? The other involves the true meaning of cure — cure for anything. It is so often said, "I went to Dr. Jones and he cured me." Nothing could be further from the truth. No matter how many years a doctor's gone to school, no matter how many college degrees he may have, a doctor can cure only one person — HIMSELF. It's important that a person understand that only he can cure himself of anything!

It's the individual and that individual's body chemistry that cure disease. In doing this, the person must take note that he's physical, structural, mental, and spiritual, and that each facet plays a part in the cure. His physician or clinician can only bring to his attention some of the basic Laws of God concerning health. Unfortunately, many clinicians aren't sufficiently aware of these Laws, even though they're honest and sincere, and try their hardest.

Although I'm a clinician, I've no intention of treating anyone for cancer or any other disease. I'm even more than a clinician — I'm a teacher. My purpose in writing this book is, therefore, educational: I hope it'll instruct you in God's Laws of natural good health — and particularly in those concerning malignancy (cancer) so that you can have a body free of this dreaded affliction. I call unto Yahweh — "I am that I am" — to bless this publication and send it forth to those who have the wisdom and need to use it.

True Early Signs of Cancer:

The true early signs of cancer are the signs of inadequate protein metabolism:
- Gas in the stomach or bowel
- Sudden weakness of the eyes
- Tired feeling most of the time
- Muscle weakness and cramps — first in the back, then in the chest
- Extreme mental depression
- Sudden change in hair texture or color
- Development of various hernias (only in slow-growing tumors)
- Confusion — difficulty in making even simple decisions

I had cancer for more than 3 years before the true nature of the problem ever dawned on me. At the height of the cancer I supposedly had about two months to live. If I'd not discovered God's Laws concerning cancer and applied them diligently, I'd not be here to share this information.

With few exceptions by the time one discovers cancer it has been with that person for a long time;

this was my situation. Now that I really know all the true early signs of cancer, I also know that I was being warned many months before my case became clinical. From time to time, I noticed belching just a little gas, but didn't give it much thought — just supposed I'd eaten a little too much. Eventually, I began to pass gas from the bowel, a little at first and finally so much that it was embarrassing to me and also my family."

My First Warning

My hobby was antique automobiles. On one trip the family made to Colorado in our 1923 Cadillac, I noticed that at dusk I found it difficult to read the road signs. I had to be right up to them before they became legible. I still didn't have the good sense even to suspect I had cancer, and didn't give the matter much more thought until 2 months later, when I was showing some slides to the Antique Automobile Club. I couldn't seem to get the pictures in focus. I thought I had damaged my camera, but the club members said the pictures were very clear and that I'd better have my eyes checked. Finally, I gave in and made an appointment with the ophthalmologist for an eye examination. To my horror, he prescribed trifocals. My protests went for naught, and I could see my pictures and road signs much better.

My Second Warning

Things went on about the same for several months, until I began to notice that if I sat in one position for more than 20 minutes, I'd have muscle aches, particularly in the back. My physician finally gave me a muscle relaxant, after I'd visited him several times with the same complaint. I was still too naïve to suspect cancer. The medication didn't help much, and in another month or so I began to have pains in my chest; this, of course upset me considerably, and I rushed to the physician once more. Over the next few months several electrocardiograms were made and nothing out of the ordinary showed; it couldn't, because the pain was from the chest muscles — a frequent sign of cancer — but as usual, I was oblivious to the true early-warning signs.

My Third Warning Went Unheeded

A long, long horrible period of mental depression followed — another true warning sign that cancer was rearing its ugly head. I went to the physician again and practically begged for help, asking for an antidepressant drug or anything that'd help alleviate this chronic, severe depression. By this time, he was fed up with me and my complaints. He sat me down and carefully explained that there was nothing wrong with me. My heart was better than his, and it was high time that I stopped worrying about it; after all, it was only in my mind!

As cancer progresses, it gives off a toxin that makes one extremely depressed, and there's a feeling of impending death a good part of the time. Gradually, during the entire 3 years of early cancer growth in my body, I became weaker and weaker. By this time I knew something tragic was taking place, but didn't know what, and still didn't have any suspicion that it might be cancer.

My job, the work I loved so much, became distasteful; I wanted to give it up and start a new profession — anything to attempt regaining an interest in life. After all the many years of college training for a job I loved to do, I was seriously contemplating junking it all. After 8 years of clinical practice and research I found myself ready to throw in the towel. It was a terrible feeling to be so sick and not be able to understand why or put a name on it. My thinking became fuzzy, unclear and irrational.

My Fourth Warning

At this time of my fourth warning I still had not an inkling in my mind what the culprit might be. During these many months of severe depression my hair began showing signs of lifelessness, becoming brittle and coarse; I was losing some, and what was left was fast becoming gray.

My Fifth Warning

My fifth warning also escaped my attention. Also, at this time, I developed a hernia, typical of a person with malignancy, since the malignancy is accompanied by muscle deterioration."

My Sixth Warning

By this time I was feeling so bad that I reluctantly returned to my physician. He finally admitted that there might be something wrong and sent me off to an internist. After the passing of 3 month's time, during which the Beard Anthrone Cancer test had proved extremely positive and I'd undergone many other tests and diagnostic procedures including X-rays, the internist finally suggested biopsies of my pancreas, liver, and intestines. He suspected that these operations would reveal cancer. Although the biopsies weren't performed, the physician's suspicions were correct.

My wife was privately told not only that I had tumors in all three organs, but also that in the doctor's opinion I had no more than 18 months to live. And though I'd begun to suspect the worst, another month passed before I myself learned of all the facts. Meanwhile, the chief surgeon in our locale had ruled out full-scale surgery because he thought I was in such bad shape that I wouldn't make it off the operating table alive. My wife had been told to take me home and get our affairs in order as promptly as possible, for it wouldn't be long before I'd pass away.

Ironically, although I 'd been doing cancer research for several years, it never occurred to me that I could have it myself. I was just like thousands of people who think it can happen to someone else — but not to them. Only the cancer victim can understand the fear and despair that finally overwhelmed me. These feelings hit me harder probably than they would have the average person, because I'd been studying and researching the details of cancer and had a firsthand insight into that horror of horrors.

Since early childhood, I experienced a deep and abiding interest in all facets of medicine and spent much of my life studying anything and everything I could find in the field. I spent two and one-half-years with the military medics and 14 years working my way through college in hospitals, doing everything from running electrocardiograms to assisting in surgery — viewing firsthand the complete gamut of medical practices and witnessing the tragic decline and ultimate death of hundreds of hopeless cancer victims.

With this great deal of knowledge about the medical community's various approaches to cancer I knew that, in spite of all the propaganda fed to the general public about success rates with certain treatments, there were actually few people who survived the medical establishment's chemicals, surgical procedures, and radiation treatments. I didn't want to be another one of its statistics. As soon as I realized my true situation, I decided not to take any new patients and prayed that I'd be granted time to complete the work with the patients already under my care. It took me about 2 weeks to overcome the terrific shock and to wrestle with my fate. After days of intensive thought and prayer, I decided not to accept the fate of an early death. Instead, I accepted life and my duty to seek out God's Laws concerning cancer and, if possible, apply them to myself and teach them to others.

My doctors had considered performing surgery on me, but they didn't think I'd make it through the operation, I was so near death. God, in His infinite wisdom, had another path for me. Not being able to have surgery turned out to be a great blessing, but, of course, I didn't see it that way at the time. The only thing I could do then was regulate my diet. My life hung in such a delicate balance (another blessing) that I could clearly feel the effect of each food I ingested. If I ate wrong foods, I could easily tell it by the way I felt.

As time passed, I realized one of the basic laws of cancer: Wrong foods caused the malignancy to grow, while proper foods allowed natural body defenses to work and the malignancy to be absorbed a little; this is one reason some people can live so long with cancer, while others succumb very quickly. Through a process too long to describe here, I worked out the relationship of enzymes, minerals, and co-enzymes, as well as proper detoxification procedures.

By the time I started my program, I was in bad shape, extremely depressed, with nothing seeming to work out well. I had a feeling of impending death most of the time, was always tired, and became completely exhausted at the slightest effort. The cancer had eaten into the nerve connections to my heart, causing rapid pulse rates and irregular beating. My cancerous pancreas was so damaged and enlarged that I had hypoglycemia and was going into insulin shock several times a day. My liver also was cancerous and enlarged. I couldn't eat much, as I was so nauseated. My intestines were so laden with cancer that I was in constant pain. I'll have scars for a long time to come.

When I finally worked out the total nutritional support program, I thought everything would be wonderful and I'd recover without further difficulties. But I had still another lesson to learn. Recovery can be worse than the disease itself. I not only had to destroy the cancer, but I had to rebuild a badly damaged body.

At first I was anxious to destroy the cancer as quickly as possible, but found that the toxic poisons made me extremely ill. I had to learn how to be sure the cancer was dissolving, but not too fast. At the proper rate one would feel sick, but not violently ill. As the body absorbs the cancer, it overloads the blood and liver with toxic poisons, making one feel constantly sick; this, for me, lasted about 8 months after the cancer growth was stopped. All the while the mental depression remains and the diet leaves you with cravings. One has been accustomed to all the tasty "junk" and it's hard to give it up forever.

As I began to get over the "goopy" sick feeling, I noticed that I'd have a good day when I felt wonderful, then several bad days when I felt "goopy" sick again. I enjoyed the good days so much that the bad ones seem much worse than they really were. I finally realized how sick I'd been.

About the time I was having a few more goods days than bad, I started having muscle cramps — bad ones. This condition went on for a minimum of 9 months, and often much longer, while I was rebuilding muscle protein taken out of the tissue during the early stages of the cancer. This stage was similar to the severe growing pains I'd experienced as a child or youth.

There's a pot of gold at the end of the rainbow — one's good health! If all the steps have been faithfully carried out, one's body is in better condition than ever before in many cases. That wasn't true in my case, at least it hasn't been yet. Although my "incurable" cancer is cured, it did a lot of damage, and it was 5 years before I was free of pain and felt really good. Nevertheless, I was given years of precious, productive living. And if you can first find hope and then health through Metabolic Medicine, I'll not have lived in vain.

Pancreatic Cancer Study

The most outstanding study in medical history is of pancreatic cancer. At the request of Robert A. Good, Ph.D., M.D., former president of Memorial Sloan-Kettering Cancer Center of New York City, Nick Gonzalez, a medical student, reviewed thousands of Dr. Kelley's patient's records selecting 22 patients with pancreatic cancer. Although Dr. Kelley had many more patients who were diagnosed with pancreatic cancer, only these 22 met the rigid standards required in this study: i.e., biopsy diagnosed at a major medical institution.

Dr. Good requested this study, which is called a numerator/denominator. In this study, a single form of cancer was chosen. Gonzalez chose pancreatic cancer since the five-year survival rate in orthodox medicine is virtually zero.

In this study a total of 22 Kelley pancreatic cancer patients properly diagnosed by the orthodox medical community were broken down into three groups, based on their level of following Kelley's protocol. The median survival of the three groups is:

Unit One: Ten patients never followed the protocol; average survival 67 days.

Unit Two: Seven patients followed the protocol partially; average survival 233 days.

Unit Three: Five patients followed Dr. Kelley's protocol completely achieved an average of 9 years survival.

In fact, all 5 were still alive at the time the study was made except one patient who had died (of Alzheimer's) after 11.5 years, cancer free.

Conclusion

For over 37 years our researchers have had the integrity, discipline and stamina to thoroughly investigate the parameters of the disease process commonly known as cancer. They have addressed this issue, a most serious one of our times with honesty, integrity, openness and determination that befits the intelligence and position of scientific researchers.

The highest honor a true scientific researcher can ever attain has been attained — that is rejection and condemnation by the Establishment. This honor comes to few in the academic or scientific community. No higher honor can be bestowed upon a mere mortal. These brave researches stand tall beside the great of civilization, such as Galileo, Louis Pasteur and Gregor Mendel.

Unfortunately, the orthodox and alternative clinicians, doctors, and researchers for well over the past 100 years have been in serious **SCIENTIFIC ERROR,** when addressing cancer. Yes, many of these individuals have observed one small parameter of cancer, but have completely missed the understanding of what cancer is. Many of the alternative researchers and practitioners have fallen into the same scientific error as the Orthodox researchers. More unfortunately, the orthodox researchers and practitioners have, even with their unlimited funding, fallen into complete and total Scientific error when addressing cancer.

1. **They see a malignant tumor mass and in <u>total scientific error</u> call it a "cancer." It is nothing of the sort. This is exposing their total ignorance of cancer. A malignant tumor mass is a malignant tumor mass, and in no way can an intelligent scientist call it cancer.**
2. **Cancer is a simple failure of one's own pancreas to produce adequate activated pancreatin and deliver it to the site of a stimulated (activated) normal trophoblast cell (pre-placenta cell). This happens to each of us thousands of times every day. Pancreatin seeks and searches out all manner of defective cells, bruises and pre-placental tissue cells.**
3. **These defective cells are digested by the activated pancreatin. The white cells then pick up this goopy mess and carry it to the LIVER by way of the bloodstream and lymph system. This mess has to wait its turn to enter the liver to be eliminated. Most doctors and cancer victims alike, are so dumb they expect the liver to do this without their help — and for the most part, the liver must accomplish this task in spite of their hindrance.**
4. **All systems of both the orthodox and alternative medical communities, in total ignorance dealing with malignant tumor masses are accounted for in Metabolic Medicine's paradigm; this is noted on page 11. The success rates of these most unscientific procedures range from 4 to at most 30%. Their few successes are accomplished by accident and in total ignorance of metabolic principles.**
5. **Few sincere, naïve, ignorant individuals in honesty and dedication want to help the CANCER VICTIM. However, they do not comprehend what cancer is and by hit or miss, stumble onto one small parameter of Metabolic Medicine's paradigm.**
6. **Most individuals associated with the diabolical CANCER RACKET do not want and will not allow the proper treatment of cancer to be known or used. They enlist the aid of the political, legal and medical Establishments. It is their objective to so deceive CANCER**

VICTIMS that they will run as fast as they can to the doctor.

7. **In their deceptive schemes, these Establishment con artists expect and demand that we cancer victims voluntarily beg the medical communities to plunder us and take all our assets in blind, false hope of receiving proper and adequate treatment. What little success is forthcoming is by accident and in total ignorance.**

Cancer victims have a failure of the pancreas for at least 2 years before a malignant tumor mass develops to a point that the physician becomes aware of their condition. Although these victims felt that something was wrong for several months and have often gone to the physician for help, with very little improvement noted.

When pancreatic failure progresses to a point wherein a malignant tumor mass—a false placenta—is found, in ignorance and scientific error, the physician calls this malignant tumor mass CANCER.

The diagnostic evaluation tools developed by the unscientific scientific community — that is, biopsy, scans, blood tests, X-rays, etc., are so crude it is unbelievable. By the time these crude procedures are used, it is most often too late for any effective therapeutic procedure. Remember the medical communities never, address CANCER, only malignant tumor masses.

Researchers of the College of Metabolic Medicine® developed a simple, effective and inexpensive Self-Examination Procedure for pancreatic failure in the mid-1960's. The Establishment for obvious reasons has suppressed this Self-Examination Procedure. The procedure is carefully outlined on page 17.

This Pancreas Self-Examination Procedure should be used once a year to alert one to possible pancreatic failure. This simple Self-Examination could put the National Cancer Institute and the American Cancer Society out of business within a few months.

All persons who have Cancer will die from starvation if they are not killed before——usually by their physician.

William Donald Kelley, D.D.S., M.S.
Administrator
College of Metabolic Medicine

SECTION II

CANCER CURE SUPPRESSED

SURGERY - CANCER

The next time you go to SURGERY remember Dr. Morton
When you are told you have CANCER remember Dr. Kelley.

ANOTHER TIME - ANOTHER PLACE
ANOTHER MAJOR MEDICAL ADVANCEMENT
ANOTHER DENTIST

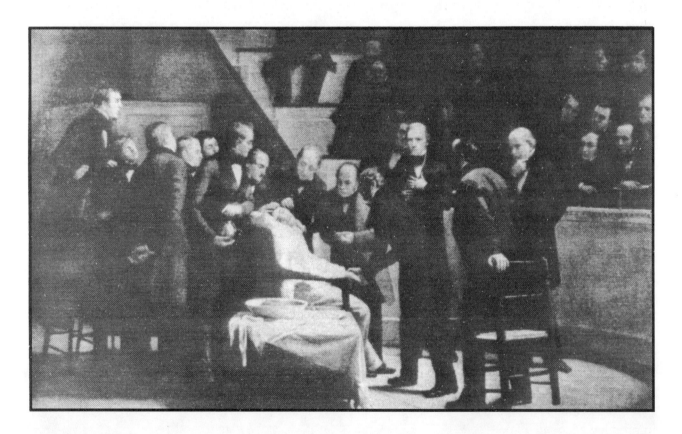

Hinckley's:
Painting of surgeons using dentist Dr. Morton's discovery of General Anesthesia on their patients. First demonstrated to the Medical Community by Dr. Morton on 16 October 1846 at Massachusetts General Hospital, thus opening the way for modern surgery. Courtesy of The Countway Library, Rare Books and Special Collections, Harvard Medical School Library, Boston.

CANCER CURE SUPPRESSED

There is not <u>ONE</u> doctor in the world today who treats cancer! Historically, we are repeating the same lesson we learned in 1930.

DR. KELLEY'S CANCER QUESTION

A diabetic going untreated will destroy his liver, kidneys, and lungs, develop a gangrenous limb and go blind. The physician who performs a liver, lung, or kidney transplant is not treating diabetes. The physician who amputates the gangrenous limb is not treating diabetes. The physician who prescribes a "Seeing-Eye-Dog" is not treating diabetes. The physician who prescribes insulin is not treating diabetes. The diabetic who gives himself insulin and changes his diet is properly treating his own diabetic condition.

The cancer victim going untreated will die a horrible, painful death. The orthodox physician who uses surgery, radiation or chemotherapy is not treating cancer. The alternative "doctor" who prescribes herbs, shark cartilage, black salve, laetrile, vitamins, etc. is not treating cancer. The Chinese doctor who prescribes 6 cockroaches and 3 grasshoppers daily is not treating cancer. These items may help something else in one's body, but will not properly treat one's cancer.

Even should these "quacks" prescribe pancreatic enzymes for the cancer victim, they are not treating cancer.

The cancer victim must treat himself by taking a safe, effective, uncontaminated form of **PANCREATIN** in adequate dosages and by changing his diet.

The "quacks" of our society are neither permitted to treat cancer, should they choose to, nor do they know how. The "quacks" of our society are only permitted to treat malignant tumors and one's purse.

The great charlatans of our civilization, like Wm. Rockefeller with his snake oil, P. T. Barnum with his circus, Barney Cornfield with his investment and insurance schemes, must look down from heaven or up from hell, green with envy and jealousy. They must beg God for a chance to be a modern-day physician.

By the time you and/or your physician discover a malignant tumor mass, you have had cancer for 2 or more years. You have to face the truth that cancer is nothing more than the failure of your pancreas to produce adequate pancreatin and your body to deliver it to the site of an injury or stimulated defective cell.

Cancer victims do not have to be a party to their own plunder and murder. They must properly treat their own cancer, as they are the only ones who can. They must embark on a "Do-It-Yourself" program.

Cancer victims want someone else to do it for them; however that is impossible, for only the victim themselves can properly treat their own cancer.

For the time being, it is not illegal to treat yourself. How long will the Establishment permit it? Only God knows.

Those who are wise enough to realize wealth is not determined in silver, gold or diamonds should consider obtaining a supply of pancreatin. Health is also an important asset.

In 1900 only 1 American in 8,000 had cancer in his lifetime. In the 37 years since I cured myself of terminal pancreatic cancer and guided some 33,000 cancer victims to health, the **CANCER RATE** has increased from 1 in 5 to, as you read this, 1 **in 2.** And the cancer industry calls this progress against cancer—the lie, the big lie. The war on cancer is the plundering war of our peoples, not a war on cancer.

DIABETES

A young man, Ernest Scott, getting his MS from Rockefeller University in 1911, discovered insulin; this was his Thesis. All the great scientists could not figure out what insulin was or how to obtain it. It is a most interesting story of God's direction of Scott. He presented it to the Rockefeller University of Chicago and submitted the completed document and his mentor professor was to publish it. The mentor changed it "for publication" and did not publish it. However, the University still has Scott's original thesis.

Scott became interested in diabetes while teaching in high school the year before he started his graduate studies. One of his high school students, a football player, did not show up for practice. Scott went to the student's home, where he learned the boy had just been told he had diabetes. In 1911 and until the late 1920's and early 1930's, diabetes was always a death sentence (even as cancer is today). The young man said: "What's the use of playing football? I'll soon die."

The next year Scott, as a graduate student in physiology, was doing experiments on dogs that had had their pancreas removed or tied off. When the <u>Diener</u> (a German word for laboratory assistant-animal-attendant employee of the university) quit because of the fly problem and sticky urine puddles from these dogs, Scott immediately figured out that the urine had high concentrations of sugar. This conclusion led Scott to discover insulin and separate the insulin secretions from the pancreatin; no one had ever done that before.

Scott went on to Columbia University to get his Ph.D. and remained on staff for years. His doctoral dissertation was the development of the Standard Blood Test for Diabetes. The story is too long to go into here, however, Eli Lilly Co. was only a name on a garage until the 1930's, when they started producing insulin by stealing Scott's 1911 insulin process.

In 1997 the Eli Lilly Trust Fund was the richest in the world, exceeding the Ford Foundation for the first time. The medical Establishment used the pancreatin part of Scott's research, patented it, then gave this monopoly to the Viobin Company, a subsidiary of the A.H. Robins Pharmaceutical Co.

Essentially, Viobin has the worldwide monopoly for the production of pancreatin, just as Lilly has the worldwide monopoly for insulin.

The medical Establishment gave the 35 million-dollar plant, having never been used, that Oscar Meyer made to go into competition with Viobin when Viobin's patent ran out in August 1983, to the Viobin Company for $5 million in one of their typical procedures.

- All pancreatin comes from one company, Scientific Protein Laboratories.
- All vitamins come from Hoffmann-LaRoche Inc., Nutley, New Jersey.
- All minerals come from Eastman Kodak Co., Rochester, New York.

Thus, from the beginning of time diabetes was a death sentence, until in 1911 when Professor Scott discovered and documented the cause and cure of diabetes. All physicians had only treated the results of diabetes, such as heart, liver and kidney damage, gangrene and blindness, but not diabetes. Everything went along the same as usual, diabetic patients dying, until the 1920's when Scott developed and standardized the blood test for diabetes. During this period, the medical Establishment in their pompous ignorance and diabolical greed murdered Scott's wife and only son with the use of Biological agents. The Eli Lilly Co. was given the sole monopoly for the manufacture and sale of insulin by the Big Establishment, which controls all monopolies. Lilly's problem was, they could not make insulin. Therefore by stealth, deceit and conspiracy, a Lilly conspirator confiscated Scott's procedures and technique for production of insulin.

The big Jew Sanhedrin's mdical Establishment Mafia then forced Sir Frederick Banting, a biologist, to accept a Doctor of Medicine degree that he did not want and in which he had no interest. Next the Establishment gave the Nobel Prize to Banting (an honorable man) and Best (not so honorable) to cover up Lilly's theft of Scott's scientific discovery. Thus, the Big Establishment conferred credibility upon Eli Lilly and Company. Lilly has had the monopoly on insulin ever since, making hundreds of millions of dollars down through the years.

So it is today. The physician only treats malignant tumor masses, blood and immune system failures, by what in the vernacular is called the slash (surgery), burn (radiation and poison (chemotherapy) procedures. Any physician who tries to use any other procedures, regardless of scientific data on its effectiveness, are subject to the following hazards:

1. He is immediately stripped of his license to practice medicine; and/or is
2. Thrown in jail for at least one year; and/or is
3. Run out of the country (usually to Mexico); and/or is
4. Killed. (I have been poisoned 3 times and shot at once.

For the time being cancer victims must treat their own cancer. Legally, they must also allow the physician to treat the results of CANCER and plunder and frequently kill the victims. (Dr. Kelley's Pancreas Self-Examination Procedure® for early detection of pancreatic failure is carefully outlined in Chapter II.)

I bring this message to you for several reasons. First, to remind you how desperately ill cancer victims become and how easy it is for me to tell them what is needed to regain their health and also how exceedingly difficult it is for them to do it. Cancer victims must give up any hope they might have that their orthodox or alternative treatments can be more than 20% successful. Although their honest physicians tell them this, it remains hard to let go of the faintest glimmer of hope. The discipline necessary to do our Metabolic Program is a high hurdle for all cancer victims.

For example, a young man, Scott Stirling, a seriously ill cancer victim, came to my little office (a 3-room shack) in Grapevine, Texas. At this point the Metabolic Nutritional Supplements were pure and uncontaminated. The medical Establishment was livid with me personally and deceived themselves that I was a health food nut and no threat to their 750 billion-dollar a year CANCER racket of plunder and murder.

Scott, of course, like other cancer victims, had to work hard to reverse the progression of his terminal illness. Our Metabolic Paradigm was, and is, as true as gravity. Like other scientists before me who found the truth down through history, the Establishment tries with all their diabolic schemes and tricks to destroy the truth. Truth is a most difficult thing to destroy. If the Establishment cannot destroy truth, they then make an all-out effort to control and profit from it, as above in the case of insulin.

I would be doing you, the reader, a disservice should I fail to tell you the whole story. Hope is a most powerful healing tool. However, false hope, dishonest and deceitful, deliberate misrepresentation is wickedness to the point of sin. Cancer victims obtain more than their share of FALSE HOPE from the Establishment's orthodox medical community. When cancer victim discern this in their fight for life and abandon orthodox medicine, they are devastated. At this point, cancer victims in their search for health, understanding and TRUTH fall prey to the ruthless wolves of alternative medicine and health care. Both orthodox and alternative health professionals are not necessarily wicked, but are all ignorant and unscientific in their treatment of cancer.

Cancer victims should take careful note that the support organizations of these plunderers also derive their income as leeches from the ignorance abounding in the cancer misinformation mania of our civilization. From the American Cancer Society, the National Cancer Institute, the various Aids organizations, to the Cancer Control Society, to the Cancer Clinics in Mexico, a lot of money and misinformation changes hands with little TRUTH or HELP.

I am taking the liberty of listing briefly some of the techniques used by the Establishment since the 1960's to **SUPPRESS THE CANCER CURE,** to maintain their control and further their annual 750-billion-dollar a year "Cancer Racket." My trials by Establishment experiences have been extensive in the field of medicine and particularly the area of CANCER. Your first reaction to this may be to stop here and mark this off as the ranting and ravings of a religious right-wing NUT. However, you do have a brain, no matter how washed and laundered and programmed it may be. You can still think and reason and know right from wrong, TRUE from FALSE, and the ring of righteousness from the thud of wickedness.

What I will communicate to you in the following pages is:
- The medical Establishment does not want a CURE FOR CANCER and absolutely will not permit a CURE for any reason, at any cost.
- CANCER is a simple dysfunction to properly treat.
- CANCER VICTIMS must treat the cancer themselves as the physicians in our society are not permitted to treat CANCER, only the effects of cancer.
- It is most difficult to CURE your own cancer.
- The Establishment deceives you with a multitude of tricks.
- It takes dedication and hard work to follow the correct Metabolic Program
- The Orthodox Medical Community plunders cancer victims. A major part of the dread that cancer victims and their families is not only the fear of physical suffering with little hope for a cure, but also the financial destruction that they face.
- Cancer Victims are used and abused Establishment research "animals." The physical torture they have to undergo from surgery, radiation, and chemotherapy has been described by one of my recent patients as worse than the tortures of he suffered in a Japanese concentration camp in World War II.

While Scott was sitting in my office getting his Metabolic Nutritional Program, the Establishment was continuing their relentless attack on the scientific paradigm, which I advanced. This attack has been ongoing since I published the scientific treatise in a little 38-page booklet, *ONE ANSWER TO CANCER*, in December 1967. Early in 1970 the Establishment had obtained a copy and went berserk, promptly throwing me in jail. Using their Establishment Media, *The Fort Worth Star Telegram,* the usual smear job belched forth to warn the public of the villain in their midst and to beware of "QUACKS."

This ruthlessness and lawlessness has gone on since the "Garden," which I thoroughly understand from history, as well as personal experience. I am reminded of another dentist, Dr. William T.G. Morton, who first discovered general anesthesia and the wicked ways in which he was treated by the Establishment, even having to suffer the theft of his paradigm and being discredited until long after his death. Even today the Establishment tries to discredit him.

THE ESTABLISHMENT

Many are allowed to rant and rave about the conspiracy in the medical Establishment and governmental agencies, but none are allowed to be truthful and point out or define who the Establishment is. To some, it is a vague somebody or group somewhere out there, who are the bad guys; to others, it is not socially acceptable or politically correct to TELL, if they know.

We politely refer to the ENEMY WITHIN as the Establishment. We all know it exists in all areas of civilization: political, economic, legal, education, health, media, and religion. The inclusive extent and wickedness of the Establishment is beyond the mental capacity of one to conceive and comprehend. The overthrow of our government and our institutions is complete. This overthrow of our institutions has not been with guns but with words, bribes, stealth, and acts of deceit.

When Scott was in my office, I had just gone through every court in Texas and the U.S. Supreme Court seeking my First Amendment Constitutional rights. However, the Establishment controls the courts and said I had no 1st amendment right or freedom of speech, freedom of press, or freedom to publish a scientific paper. In fact the Establishment was so angry and livid, they claimed the book was practicing medicine on anyone who read it. "Dr. Kelley is a clear and present danger to society" (translates: Establishment interests). Only Justice William O. Douglas dissented (1971). I am not allowed to have a copy of the book.

Double Jeopardy

The Establishment was so livid and upset, they forced the Texas State Board of Dental Examiners to remove my dental license for 5 years on the same charges. Double jeopardy is also unconstitutional.

Like Scott, almost everyone who visited me or followed this 38-page booklet, recovered in about 6 months. During this period of time, if it took longer than 6 months the victim was not following the booklet or continued with chemotherapy and/or radiation.

To say this scenario upset the local oncologists throughout the country was the understatement of the century. Among cancer victims this booklet spread like a wild forest fire. Many cancer victims never visited me, but nevertheless recovered and went on their way to health.

Of course, this result was reported to the local state medical boards, which in turn reported to the medical Establishment.

Texas State Agencies

At this point the Establishment was in a first class tizzy. They engaged in the practice of sending the police to sit outside of my little 3 room shack of an office, stopping each one of my dental patients, trying to get a confession that they were coming to visit me for treatment of cancer, not for a visit to the dentist.

Grapevine, Texas, the site of the dental office, was 4-5 miles north of the Dallas/Ft. Worth Airport. Counselees flying into D/FTW would rent a car and drive to my office. The police would take down the rental car's license, then go to the rental agency and get the names and addresses of counselees. In addition to giving the information to the Establishment, the police would send it to the hometown of the counselee, so their local police could keep surveillance on them. Many entrapment tricks both in Texas and hometowns were used frequently.

Another First

The Establishment got into such a frenzy they engaged the Texas State Comptroller to illegally do their dirty work. They were determined to stop me at all costs. The Establishment sent to my little shack an agent of the Comptroller. It did not bother me a bit. In fact I offered to help the Comptroller. The Comptroller decided that I owed the sovereign State of Texas several thousands of dollars in sales taxes I should have collected on the food and vitamins being sold to counselees. CHANGING THE LAW RETROACTIVELY, a good ol' Establishment trick he learned from the IRS, who practice it routinely, when needed to control or destroy a person.

The state legislature specifically by law exempted sales tax on food and vitamins. The Comptroller, Bob Bullock (later to become Lt. Governor) said he made a specific arbitrary ruling for me [by Establishment's orders]. I just ignored him. Being challenged, the Comptroller got nasty and sent his henchmen to threaten me. I told them, "I'll make a deal with you. You can pay for a clerk to collect it for you. I only work for myself. Or, you can set up a card table outside my front door and collect the taxes yourself. I'll even let you store your card table inside my office overnight. You'd better have a beach umbrella, because sitting outside in the Texas sun gets hot." Last December I received a Christmas card from Lt. Governor & Mrs. Bullock.

Not too long after we moved to a tiny town of 200 in Winthrop, Washington. The Establishment was enraged to a point of hate and action. One wintry night our home was burned to the ground. All was lost including the older stored medical records and our pets.

During this period no Establishment trick was overlooked to stop me. The Establishment-controlled Federal agency, Internal Revenue Service, used all its reserve tricks, and like the Texas Comptroller, made up several new rules in their attempt to stop me. I guess I was too dumb to let it bother me and went on my way helping as many people as God would send.

All-out Establishment War of Revenge

From late 1979 through to this date the Establishment has been in an insane tizzy. No deceit, no lie, no trick, no bribe, no MURDER, no use of "the badder and baddest people" were overlooked and used to the fullest extent of their creative diabolic intent and actions. In their war on me they attacked on all fronts and areas to the full fury of their capacity. They did several things at the same time. Many too horrible to write about; I will mention some that were all going on at the same time. The battles became intense with the Hollywood Actor Steve McQueen.

Steve McQueen

Early in 1980 after he had stopped, within 6 months, the growth of his (McQueen's) own cancer tumors, his body had encapsulated the dead liver tumor and several smaller masses.

McQueen felt well and demanded that the unsightly bulge on his right side and little nodule on the left side of his neck be surgically removed. I was against this surgery at the time but McQueen insisted.

Fatal Mistake

McQueen frequently called me on my FBI-tapped telephone. In one call McQueen made to me, he stated in his famous hero's voice, "I'm going to blow the lid off this Cancer Racket." This threat of course, freaked out the cancer Establishment. The FBI then leaked it to the National Enquirer. This exposure was to discredit me. McQueen was then constantly watched and harassed by the FBI, CIA and the media.

McQueen Murder

During the surgery the skin over the liver was cut open and the encapsulated, dead tumor fell out on the operating table. After surgery McQueen had a talk with me. During the night a government agent came into his room, posing as a physician on duty and injected McQueen with a blood-clotting medication, which was the cause of his death.

THE ESTABLISHMENT INFILTRATION OF THE KELLEY PROGRAM

Movie actor Steve McQueen had completely cured his own CANCER using our Metabolic Program and had made plans to expose and "blow the lid off the cancer racket"; before he could accomplish this, he was murdered as only the Establishment can do it with all the fanfare and news media to destroy my program. When this failed, the Establishment's next plan was to send a mole or infiltrator into the Kelley organization so that as close a call as the McQueen episode could never happen again.

A Cornell medical student, Gonzalez, who had failed after his second year in medical school, was wandering in and out of the unorthodox medical community, looking for help for his own mental instability and illness. During this fruitless search Gonzalez stumbled onto the Kelley Program, which he mentioned to his psychiatrist.

125

With the help of his psychoanalyst, Colter Rule, M.D. and wife Betty Gessels, M.D. (high level Establishment members in NYC), Gonzalez and a major faction of the Establishment forced Robert A. Good, Ph.D., M.D., President of Memorial Sloan-Kettering Cancer Center/Institute, to sponsor Nicholas J. Gonzalez' review of Kelley's records and expose Kelley as a Quack. This project, being most important to the Establishment, led Cornell Medical School to eventually give Gonzalez an unearned M.D. degree.

The infighting of the Medical Establishment over this project forced the most renowned medical researcher of all history to be fired and dismissed from Sloan-Kettering and shipped out to Oklahoma City. The Establishment gave the green light to Gonzalez to carefully investigate the Kelley program and get the information to expose me as a fraud. This backfired on the Big Establishment as the second communication from Gonzalez to Good after Gonzalez reviewed the first 139 of thousands of records in my possession showed.

Robert A. Good, M.D., Ph.D.
2 September
Medical Research Foundation
Oklahoma Allergy Clinic
50 N.E. 13th Street
Oklahoma City, Oklahoma.

Dear Dr. Good,

I hadn't meant to write you so soon again, but I've just finished sifting through the first 139 of Dr. Kelley's patient records and found the initial results interesting enough to pass on my findings. While I intend to concentrate on the cancers we discussed — pancreatic, colon, lung, perhaps breast — I've included all the initial results just for interest's sake.

Again, as I wrote in my first letter to you, I do not yet have the actual biopsy reports or other lab data documenting the diagnosis, but I have found Dr. Kelley does keep information regarding how the tumors were diagnosed.

I found these results, particularly for pancreatic, quite intriguing. His overall survival rate for all cancer in this first group is 93% — and I have found, going through Dr. Kelley's records, virtually all of his patients have advanced disease. Many have come to him <u>because</u> <u>no</u> <u>further</u> <u>conventional</u> <u>treatment</u> <u>could</u> <u>be</u> <u>offered</u>.

Sincerely, Nick

Tumor type	#Pts. on	#Deceased	#Survival times in years to present while on program.
Adenoidal	1	0	2
Adrenal	1	0	1
Basal cell	1	0	3
Bile duct	1	0	5
Bladder	2	0	5,6
Bone	2	0	5,6
Breast	30	3	1,1,1,2,2,3,3,3,4,4,4,4,4,4,4,4,4,5,5,5,5,5,6,6,7,7,8,8,8,10
Cervical	3	0	2,3,4
Choriocarcinoma	1	0	2
Colon (all advanced)	15	0	1,1,2,3,3,5,5,6,6,7,8,8,8,10,13
Ewing's sarcoma	1	1	2
Fibrous Histiocytoma	(1)	0	5
Hodgkin's	4	0	1,1,3,10
Leukemia (unclassified)	1	0	8
Leukemia, acute lymphocytic	2	0	1/2,2
Leukemia, acute myelocytic	2	0	4,5
Leukemia, chronic	1	0	1
Lung	6	2	2,3,4,6,8,8
Lymphocytic Lymphoma (unclassified)	14	1	1,1,2,2,2,3,3,4,5,5,5,5,5,13
Melanoma	5	2	1,3,4,4,6
Metastatic (adenocarcinoma)	2	0	6,6
Multiple myeloma	(2)	0	1,3
Ovarian	3	0	2,5,8
Pancreatic (4 diagnosed at exploratory)	8	0	1,3,3,4,5,7,8,8
Parotid	1	0	5 1/2
Plasmacytoma	(1)	0	9
Prostate	8	0	1/2,2,3,3,3,4,4,8
Rhabdomyosarcoma	(1)	0	4
Seminoma	1	0	5
Skin, unclassified	6	0	1,2,2,3,3,8
Small intestine	(2)	0	3,7 1/2
Stomach	2	0	4 1/2, 6
Trophoblastic	(1)	0	6
Urethal	1	0	3 1/2
Uterus	6	0	3,3,6,7,8,10

Conspiracy, Fraud, Takeover

The diabolical cult organization, SCIENTOLOGY, had several of their doctors and nurses attend my Metabolic Technician Training Seminars. They were using the Computerized Metabolic Program on their "sick Church members" with excellent results. As is the case with all divisions of the Establishment, they wanted to take over the Kelley organization. They could see millions of dollars in income and control of a whole system of medicine. They too, sent one of their "slick con artists," a Barney Cornfield type, to Dallas and announced they were to take over the organization. Just get out of the way. We're going to do Kelley a big favor, We may give him a little royalty, but most of it he must give to our 'Church.'

An Inside Job

This little experience scared my employees so badly, they went into a frenzy. They had been planning a take-over of the Kelley organizations for some time. Masterminded by my own lawyer and accountant, they got down to the business of throwing me out of my own organization and taking over.

Establishment at Work

The Establishment could not depend upon Good and Gonzalez, delay any longer, or take any more halfway measures. I was a most serious threat to their $750-Billion-a-year industry. These lawless Establishment devils went to work and:

- Poisoned (food) me 3 times to the point of grand mal seizures 3-4 times a week for 14 months;
- tried to shoot me once during this time;
- sent the usual IRS agents to do me in;
- bought off and bribed my lawyer and accountant;
- set up a takeover of the Kelley organization by employees and wife (standard Establishment procedure);
- offered Kelley $500,000 to kill a counselee; and
- caused a vitamin manufacturer of supplements Kelley often used to take all active ingredients out of Kelley Program Supplements.

Use of the Media

The media is a most useful tool for the Establishment. Two encounters of hand-to-hand battle occurred during this time by the media to brainwash the general public of the ineffectiveness and danger of the Kelley Metabolic Program

The Establishment's Tom Brokaw and his "side kick authority figure, Art Euline, M.D., a Gynecologist" did a first class smear job of discrediting me on the NBC TODAY show.

Several months later, the BBC with Prince Charles produced a real hatchet job on me. I had several contacts (friends) in England, one a former Jehovah Witness from New Zealand, and one a Mormon from the U.S. A few months before the BBC show I went to London and made the rounds of available hospital facilities from the Florence Nightingale to the City Hospitals. These backers had agreed to financially support moving the Kelley operations to England. Using the FBI-tapped phone lines, the Big Establishment both in the United States and England went into a tizzy over this and dispatched their number-one BBC documentary crew to Dallas to interview me and make a despicable TV program with Prince Charles introducing it. The program was scathing and intended to stop anyone in Europe from working with me.

Scott and several of the Kelley patients were requested by the BBC to come to Dallas for the filming at their own expense. The patients can verify how desperately ill I was at the time from the Establishment's poisoning.

ESTABLISHMENT MURDERS

The next battles with the Establishment were a series of premeditated murders by the Establishment. These murders were carried out in two stages involving several hundred cancer victims and several children with cystic fibrosis.

STAGE ONE

Fractionation

The A.H. Robins Co, like the Eli Lilly Co., was given the sole worldwide monopoly for pancreatin by the Big Establishment. Pancreatin was the only nutritional supplement used by all of the Kelley patients.

Murder, Deceit, Fraud, Murder

The first procedure used by the Establishment to put an end to me was the development of a process by which to fractionate the whole pancreatin into the various individual enzymes. In fractionating the pancreatin, they were able to remove one of the major enzymes and make it unavailable to the nutritional market. They continued to market the defective pancreatin to the unsuspecting health food market. Supplement manufacturers never knew why their products were no longer effective for a multitude of nutritional needs. When I personally informed these manufacturers, I was threatened with legal action; being aware of this, I adjusted our Metabolic Program to compensate for this fraud. I continued helping the cancer victims, but instead of a 6-month procedure the program, had to be extended for 18 to 24 months. The cost was also greatly increased.

The Establishment, by removing needed active ingredients in the raw materials sold to the companies making vitamin tablets, assumed the Kelley Program was doomed to total failure. Although I altered our Metabolic Program to compensate for this, those who now claim they have the Kelley Program and supplements are deceiving themselves and the cancer victim, for this is the state of PAN-

CREATIN and their fraudulent programs of cancer cures to date.

The chymotrypsin removed from pancreatin is now sold to manufacturers of sewer and septic tank cleaners and not available to the medical community or health food store industry.

STAGE TWO

Biological Weapons in the Cancer War

My fellow-researcher, Dr. Carol A. Morrison, found that the A.H. Robins Co. laced the pancreatin they were marketing to the medical and health supplement industries in our country with a deadly bacteria, B. cereus (Gram-positive Endospore-forming). This infection is a member of the B. anthraces (ANTHRAX) family and was totally undetectable in the human body by any known medical procedure, laboratory or biopsy, until recently. Like anthrax infection is always fatal unless properly addressed immediately. This infection is part of a wide experimental biological warfare program being conducted by the highest levels of the big diabolical Jew Sanhedrin's medical Establishment. The Establishment for several years has used this experimental biological agent.

The Establishment, which controls the U.S. governmental agencies, has several purposes in mind when infecting various parts of the population with biologicals, both natural and man-made, one objective being the destruction of the pancreas with the resulting astronomical increases in diabetes and cancer. Another goal is a form of genocide for select racial groups. Remember, the Establishment has been doing for a long time what they accuse others of doing.

National Cancer Institute

The Establishment politicians passed legislation to declare WAR on CANCER. Thus, they went to Fort Detrick and took down the U.S. Army Chemical and Biological Warfare department SIGN. They then placed two signs on the front gate of the facility: on the left, NATIONAL CANCER INSTITUTE (NCI) and on the right, WORLD HEALTH ORGANIZATION (WHO). This was and is properly ballyhooed by the Establishment media, and financed to the tune of several hundred billion dollars yearly from American taxpayers.

Mad Scientists

It is no wonder EVE was deceived in the Garden of Eden. We really cannot blame her. For even today the enemy within is deceiving us. Of course, the most evil and mad scientists of all recorded history (at Fort Detrick) never missed an hour of work or a paycheck and continued as usual. While this work is going on, Establishment politicians from their United Nations (UN) center send out teams of inspectors to make sure other nations do not develop and use biological warfare weapons. These clever and deceptive Establishment politicians play by a different set of rules than others are allowed to play by.

Heads I win, tails you lose

Human Experimental Animals

These mad scientists, using human fetal DNA material, produce new bacterial and viral infectious agents. They use and alter the DNA material from deadly bacteria and virus to successfully escape known antibiotic and antiviral treatment procedures work four objectives:

1. To obtain additional taxpayer funding and enslavement
2. To reduce the world population. (Population Act of 1981)
3. To further plunder Americans by their relief organizations: Red Cross, Feed the Starving, Save a Child Campaign, etc..
4. To give credibility to their dedicated diabolical scientific endeavors.

With these new genetic altered biological weapons are ready, now they are using various segments of our population for their "Controlled Studies." This has gone on in America since the early 1800s. The 1930s Tuskegee Syphilis Study on Blacks and the smallpox and typhus epidemics of the American Indians are examples of this highly developed skill of the Establishment, as well as the various epidemics of tuberculosis (TB) used during the last 150 years.

When America took the Philippine Islands from Spain, General Arthur MacArthur, father of General of the Armies Douglas MacArthur of World War II fame, was ordered by the political Establishment to inoculate the general population of the Philippines with live smallpox vaccine, which killed more people than the previous smallpox epidemics. Also, in 1950 the U.S. military experimented on Eskimos and Indians with radioactive drugs.

First Success

The mad scientists at the NCI and WHO, who had taken over the U.S. Army's biological facility at Fort Detrick, Maryland, finally had the success in the venture the U.S. Government spent so much of your tax money on.

AIDS—Imposed Genocide

There is absolutely no scientific evidence that this laboratory-engineered virus was present in Africa before the WHO descended upon these hapless people with their deadly AIDS-laced vaccine. The AIDS virus did not come from Africa; it **came from Fort Detrick, Maryland, U.S.A.**

Who "Invented" AIDS

It is a mind boggling revelation, which has been alleged from the beginning of the AIDS fiasco, to realize that AIDS is a diabolical, laboratory-contrived plague, imposed upon society by design and plan. The evidence is clear: The government of the U.S.A. has no intention of protecting American society from AIDS.

Hitting the Target

The mad, mad scientists at the NCI and WHO have so perfected their man-made bacteria and virus to the point of being able to select which part of the human body they want to destroy and what type of human cells they wish to target. AIDS was just one such achievement — to destroy the immune system "T" cells. Although it was their first success, it was certainly not their last.

Now they have MAD COW, man-made biologicals, to use against the brain. They also have EBOLA for liver and other organs. This biological was first tested on the American Indian children and later on natives in South America.

Cancer

Recently, one of their most accomplished biological targeted areas is the human pancreas. This is how our government can predict in advance the incidence of diabetes and Cancer. By destroying the one part of the pancreas they can increase the incidence of Diabetes. By destroying another part of the human pancreas, they have been able to produce a rapid development of all types of cancer that will take a person's life within a short period of time. This is so devastating, there is very little treatment possible — and none intended. Our government funded research for this specific type of genocide is genetically engineered biological warfare agents tagged to human fetal embryo tissue from abortions and forced upon the children and general public via mandatory vaccinations among other methods. This is based upon the ancient science of Homeopathy.

Cancer Victims

In short, the cancer victims of today face the Establishment enemy within, who are relentless and determined to plunder and kill you at any cost. "False Hope" is not my objective. To be realistic, we have two enemies, CANCER and the ESTABLISHMENT. Of course there is HOPE, you must have pancreatin and other Metabolic Nutrients to treat your cancer properly. However, you must use discernment in obtaining it and be aware of the multitude of con-artists who make claims for their products. Legally, you must allow the orthodox physician to treat your tumors. Remember he is neither allowed to treat your cancer, nor is he qualified to do so. **DO NOT TAKE ANY VACCINATIONS.** This is the standard deceptive way you are given the Establishment's biological warfare infections.

Remember

There will never be permitted the CURE for cancer, even the Scientific Kelley program until the Jew Establishment can accomplish their objectives by permitting it. Their primary goals are money and control, with a secondary objective of genocide. What big conglomerate will get the blessings of the Big Establishment? Nothing happens on the world scene that is not planned and designed by the Big Jew Establishment.

Notes on Cancer Victims

After 30 years of planning Metabolic Programs for some 33,000 counselees and developing the scientific paradigm for the PROPER CURE AND TREATMENT OF MALIGNANCY, I would like to share some of the conclusions.

First, we fall victim not only to cancer but also to the clever brainwashing of our number-one ENEMY. The mdical Establishment and the unending barrage of the conspiracy with the MEDIA and support groups such as the American Cancer Society, the National Cancer Institute, the American Medical Association and an unlimited number of organizations that make their income from the crumbs that fall from the Establishment's table.

Second, our number-two ENEMY is the simple metabolic malfunction of our pancreas, a minor enemy compared to our enemies number one and three. In our Metabolic Paradigm we find approximately 20 causes for this failure.

All successes and failures of all cancer programs are accounted for by our paradigm. It would not be a truly scientific-paradigm if it did not include **ALL CANCERS**, which it does.

Third, our number three-enemy is ourselves. It is quite a shame that Yahweh, God Almighty, gave each one of us a decent brain (heart in scriptural terms), but we do not know how to use it, as we have little, if any practice. We depend upon others (with inferior hearts) to do our thinking for us. In short, we go a-whoring after false Gods and the false idols put in front of us by our enemy number one.

Those cancer victims whom God has blessed with enough time (6 months) and who have awakened from their stupor, in self-defense, figure things out for themselves. Their discernment that their physician, their medical community, the Establishment, the MEDIA and their government with its multitude of bureaucracies have conspired in fraud, plunder and murder against them, — the SHOCK is nearly overwhelming and devastating to say the least.

Fourth, at this point, in self-preservation, cancer victims rebel and in righteous indignation, often go berserk. But at least they realize they cannot trust or depend upon the orthodox medical community or the government to protect and help them, but only deceive, plunder them and murder. Also they come to the realization that to survive they must "do it themselves" and find the answers in spite of the ESTABLISHMENT'S interference, promises and brainwashing.

Fifth, in this state of abandonment, cancer victims in ignorance and desperation become vulnerable and prey to the other vultures — the alternative medical community. The alternative medical community is composed of the most skilled CON-MEN and CON-WOMEN in our civilization, falsely deceiving, like the orthodox, that they have the answer and are persecuted scientists and promoters of truth. These despicable creatures would put ol' P. T. Barnum, Wm. Rockefeller and Barney Cornfield to shame; their techniques of deception are superb. Many of these creatures also deceive themselves and are pathological liars and psychopaths. The remainders are ignoramuses.

Somewhere along the line, cancer victims turn to Almighty God and ask for deliverance, healing and help. When God sends help, like placing this book in front of their eyes, they refuse to accept it, blaming God for their condition and finally turning from God to their own ignorance.

Sixth, my experience with cancer victims over the years has taught me a great deal about the mindset of these "do-it-yourself" survivors.

- Many choose to continue to follow all the recommendations and treatments of their orthodox physicians, while at the same time, do our Metabolic program. This is usually disastrous and only about 6% survive.

- Some Cancer Victims, after their orthodox physician tells them the treatments are not effective and no further help can be expected, start our Metabolic Program. Experience has shown that 93% of these individuals who live long enough to stay on the Metabolic Program for 12-18 months recover completely and go on to live normal useful lives.

- Often the Cancer Victim goes berserk and while accusing his orthodox and/or alternative doctor of being an ignoramus and not knowing what he is doing, ends up doing exactly the same thing. He tries to <u>play</u> <u>doctor</u> without adequate scientific understanding. This seems to be an ego builder for the Cancer Victim. However, this is not successful and in the end is usually fatal.

- Nearly everyone thinks that if a little bit of something is good, then a lot of everything is better. This results in about 9% effectiveness as well as unnecessary expense. To many, this is a fun game and entertaining. They say to themselves: "If I have to go, I might as well have a blast!"

- For those who have a great deal of wisdom and discernment along with 6 months' time, while following a Metabolic Program carefully, are almost always successful.

As with diabetes, cancer victims must always support their defective pancreas with proper diet as well as effective enzymes. They must remember, that proper enzymes are difficult to obtain and always expensive.

Seventh, many cancer victims, having been brainwashed by the Establishment, give up, believing they can never recover their health and after seriously consider SUICIDE. If they choose suicde, there are several choices they can make.

A. Go first class and be slow about it. Return to the orthodox community. Here you will have all the sympathy of the National Cancer Institute, the American Cancer Society, Hospice Inc., The American Medical Association and many others. They will brainwash you and your loved ones with "Oh, how brave and heroic you are." What a valiant fight you made!"— all the while plundering your estate and your loved ones.

B. Go to Detroit, Michigan and obtain the help of the suicide doctor, if your doctor will not give his help.

C. Go to the interstate highway and jump in front of a semi; at least this will help your lawyer send his kids to college.

Letting Go

The most difficult procedure for cancer victims is to let go of the false hope that both orthodox and alternative medicine use to control and plunder. Frequently, due to their ignorance of the simple CANCER CURE, the condition is fatal.

The programs we had developed were functional until 30 August 1986. At that time, I gave up my practice of Metabolic Counseling and unplugged my computer because of activities of employees and doctors I had trained. I would not or will not be party to the plunder, fraud and conspiracy of CANCER victims and metabolic counselees.

Any program available today in my name (or claiming to be the 'Kelley Program' or better than the Kelley Program) are frauds and those who are issuing them should be considered a danger to your being. In giving cancer victims HOPE and not <u>false hope</u>, my involvement is conditional upon giving the reader the complete story, not only of the plight of cancer victims and the Metabolic Paradigm, but the missing nutrients for cancer victims. Also, be aware of the medical Establishment's all-out effort to suppress the CANCER CURE and protect their interests. My interest is to provide a sound, reliable understanding and effective metabolic procedure to supply the required metabolic support.

My objective as a teacher is to provide you, if you choose, with the necessary data by which to live a long and useful life, never dying of cancer. I would much rather have your friends and relatives read in the obituary column — you died at age 95 from gunshot wounds inflicted by a jealous lover — NOT FROM CANCER!

Notes on Dentists

Dentists are not ignoramuses bordering on stupidity; however, you could not tell that it by their actions. Dentists have killed more adults and children since 1950 than all the wars of recorded history.

Dentists themselves have been royally conned by the Establishment. Dentists have been used as willing pawns of the Establishment to plunder and murder our civilization by their support of the Establishment's covert FLUORIDE fraud "sting" operation.

Dentists know from their required studies in biochemistry that fluoride is the most deadly poison known to mankind.

Legal Poisoning

Over half of the U.S.A. population is drinking fluoridated water, which is now linked to cancer and arthritis. "Bone cancer has been linked to fluoride in a 10-year study by the National Toxicology Program of the U.S. Department of Health and Human Services." This sensational news was disclosed in an exclusive report in *Medical Tribune,* December 28, 1989, but ignored by the mass media. Also, Procter and Gamble, the maker of Crest (a fluoride toothpaste), presented studies to the U.S. Public Health Service, showing that "fluoride tested positive as a cancer-causing agent at the lowest concentrations used." According to Charles Eliot Perkins, a research chemist sent to Germany to take charge of the I.G. Farben Chemical Industries after World War II, repeated doses of fluoride were used to make people submissive to the government. He wrote, "In the rear occiput of the left lobe of the brain, there is a small area of brain tissue that is responsible for the individual's power to resist domination. Repeated doses of fluoride will in time gradually reduce the individual's power to resist by slowly poisoning and narcotizing this area of brain tissue and make him submissive to those who wish to govern him. I was told the scheme by a German chemist who was an official of the I.G. Farben Chemical Industries and prominent in the Nazi movement of the time." (The Fact Finder, Box A Scottsdale, AZ 85352)

Oral Cancer

Oral Cancer needlessly kills 10,000 people each year. Dentists, with all their legal licenses and education, are not ignoramuses. However, their integrity has been compromised and the Establishment tightly controls them. Dentists, like physicians, are not permitted to properly treat oral cancer.

It has been increasingly apparent to the general population: Our government cannot be trusted. The Establishment has long since overthrown government and are using various bureaus and agencies to control and plunder American citizens.

The Establishment's shrewd and careful creation of "Cancer Fear," while withholding cancer cure, is a major technique for plunder and control.

CANCER ANSWERS

- Since our Government has been overthrown by the enemy for many years; and
- since our country has now been completely and totally taken over by the enemy; and
- since our enemy has planned the murder of 100 million U.S. citizens before the year 2029 by use of biological warfare agents; and
- since the government has sponsored and funded major programs that induce terminal, irreversible cancer in one out of two individuals in our civilization; and
- since the medical profession is forbidden to treat cancer in patients who have been deliberately infected by government programs, via human embryonic tissue laced with biologicals and viruses, to target one's brain, liver, lung, pancreas, breast, etc.; and
- since there is no longer a cure for cancer, only rational and proper cancer treatment procedures; and
- since it is not yet illegal (and even if it becomes so) to treat oneself in a life or death survival procedure;
- it behooves one to obtain survival knowledge, understanding and wisdom for one self and one's family.

Cancer victims must treat themselves by:
- taking a safe, effective, uncontaminated form of PANCREATIN in adequate dosages
- taking an appropriate anti-biotic to counteract the infectious biological contaminants being given to our population in a multitude of ways
- changing their diet.

Cancer victims want someone else to do it for them. However that is impossible, for only the victims can properly treat their own cancer.

Obtaining a supply of pancreatin, antibiotics and whole organic grains and beans should be considered by those who are wise enough to realize wealth is not determined in silver, gold or diamonds. Health is also an important asset.

Respectfully,

William Donald. Kelley, D.D.S., M.S.
Medical Missionary, to the most
pagan peoples on earth - Americans.

Appendix I

Medical Corps Evaluations (Circa 1982)

Dr. John Rhinehart (Medical Doctor)

"I first met Dr. Kelley 6 years ago. I'd taken a seriously-ill member of my family to him for an evaluation and a 'nutritional' program. What I got was a fascinating and provocative experience about a new way to live healthfully and a whole new concept of what physical and spiritual health is all about; this was all in addition to a nutritional program. While I did not understand at that point exactly all the ramifications of his approach, I was so intrigued that I decided to go on a program myself. Part of doing this was to test for myself whether it really was possible that Dr. Kelley had developed a method for applying his theories.

My own physical problems resolved around long-term exhaustion of what I now know as my sympathetic nervous and glandular systems. Medically, these problems encompassed several diagnoses including irritable colon and mucus colitis, severe low blood sugar, intermittent episodes of high blood pressure, depression, and erratic and low-energy patterns, commonly called 'burn-out.'

What I noticed over the years was a disappearance of all my symptoms, the return of energy, endurance, and interest, which I could count on. I knew something vitally important had happened in my body and did not quite understand how that had been accomplished. So I decided to study with Dr. Kelley, in order to find some answers to that apparent riddle. What I discovered was a simple theory that addressed an extremely sophisticated piece of machinery — our bodies — in a new and comprehensive as well as therapeutically effective,way.

Over the last two years I've incorporated the program in my practice and have seen all types of people responding well, providing they commit themselves to doing the program thoroughly. I'd also like to emphasize that the program is a dynamic and ever-developing one, so much so that the changes incorporating new knowledge make year-old programs seem like ten years of age.

Overall, I believe that Dr. Kelley's program is sparked by a special sort of genius decades ahead of its time and will be a paradigm of medical care in the future."

John Rhinehart, M.D.
Newton, CT

Dr. Douglas M. Baird (Osteopathic Surgeon)

"An open letter to my colleagues, April 1982. The prevailing orientation of the traditional medical community over the past 150 years, with regard to cancer and other degenerative disease processes, has been largely a destructive, anti-symptomatic phenomenon. Admittedly, these approaches have some absolute applications for limited, short-term therapy, but in my strong opinion, anti-symptomatic therapies have no validity in the treatment of long-term disease. What is and has been needed for some years is a major re-evaluation of the medical scientific doctrine and the establishment of a more appropriate model for the understanding of health and disease. Hopefully, this new model could redirect the investigative energies of the research community on more rewarding horizons.

I feel that the time has come from both the scientific and humanistic viewpoints, for a change in emphasis from the disease process itself to the person who has the disease and from a position of fighting against disease to one of re-establishing and preserving good health. One of the major contributors to the proposed changes in medical thought has been Dr. William Donald Kelley, a dentist by profession, who developed a self-sustaining, cohesive model, which largely explains and properly categorizes volumes of seemingly divergent scientific information, theories, observations and experiences. The key is biological individuality. Dr. Kelley's genius is in developing an entire scientific model beginning with the individual and his inherent uniqueness.

A major reorganization of thought and practice is required of the medical community to utilize the tools, which have become available as a result of his model. I have used Dr. Kelley's Metabolic Medicine program for several years and the results, I can assure you, are most gratifying."

Douglas M. Baird, D.O.
Palm Beach, FL

Dr. Sanford C. Frumker (Doctor of Dentistry)

"As a periodontist, I soon became convinced that to treat those things in the mouth that cause gum disease is only partial treatment. Based on a great deal of evidence, I was convinced that if the body of the patient was well-nourished and the machinery in the mouth was working properly the patient will not have gum tissue breakdown. As a result of this thinking over many years, I-ve taken several nutrition courses. Thanks to time spent with Dr. Roger Williams and a great deal of reading and studying, I had established specific criteria for a nutritional program. With no exception, (and that was not a program I could easily use in my practice) none of the nutrition courses satisfied my criteria.

International Health Institute's (Dr. Kelley's) program was the first program I saw that at least on paper appeared both to be practical and to fill my requirements. However, since I had been led down umpteen primrose paths by other "nutrition" programs, I was skeptical of the Metabolic Medicine program.

When, with great skepticism, I started my own Metabolic Medicine program, I felt I was in excellent health. I had only one health problem that I was aware of and that was that I had nasal polyps, which were caused by allergies. The polyps were particularly bad in winter. I couldn't breathe through my nose at all. So after having the polyps surgically removed, I was referred to an allergist. The allergist found I was allergic to dust and all dairy products. I already knew about the allergy to the dairy products because after a heavy dairy meal, my nose would completely close due to the swelling of the polyps. To control the growth of the polyps, the allergist recommended weekly "allergy shots." For two years, they worked well, and I could breathe fairly well through my nose in the winter. During the third and fourth years the allergy shots did not work as well and I had trouble breathing through my nose. During the fifth and sixth years the allergy shots did not work at all. I couldn't breathe through my nose at all in the winter and very little in the summer. My allergist now informed me the only thing that would help me was cortisone injections. Knowing the undesirable effects of cortisone, I refused. Things got bad enough that finally I had one cortisone injection.

When I began my Metabolic Medicine program, I informed Dr. Kelley of my allergy to dairy products and asked him if anything could be done to help. To my surprise Dr. Kelley said he was not at all interested in my specific allergies, but only interested in getting the body working right, so I'd not be allergic to anything. I was doubtful of Dr. Kelley and the entire program at that time.

When I filled out my Nutritional Evaluation Survey, I discovered many health normalities that I never knew existed. Filling out my survey, indeed, was an experience in self-discovery and understanding. If the information and the claims for what it indicated were correct, this was the most valuable physical examination and insight into my inner workings I'd ever experienced. However, I had grave reservations as to the truth of diagnosis made from this information and the blood test and urinalysis. Therefore, I went into the program not only skeptical, but almost with a chip on my shoulder. Based on past experiences, I felt sure I was wasting my time and money. I've now been on the program for several years. Even during the first winter, with no allergy shots, no cortisone (and no allergist), my nose was open all winter. I could breathe through my nose!

Being suspicious, I could not give the Metabolic Medicine program full credit for my feeling so good. So I went back to my Metabolic Medicine's Self-Test book and compared all the signs and symptoms with where they are now. By checking these signs and symptoms, I had an objective way of seeing what this program was doing to my internal machinery! To put it mildly, the Metabolic Medicine program has been a great success for me. My allergies are under control. I've never felt better. In addition, with the Metabolic Medicine's Self-Test book, I've been able to see objectively what's happening with me. With these objective observations of myself, with certainty, at least for me, the program is an unqualified huge success.

Now convinced, I'm offering this program to all of my dental patients. I know the program does the job and that it is what we need to get our internal machinery to do the job."

Sanford C. Frumker, D.D.S.
Cleveland, OH

Dr. Lloyd H. Price (Doctor of Optometry)

"My training as an optometrist started long before I entered Northwest Illinois Optical College in Chicago, Illinois, in 1922. As a farm boy, I had the opportunity to observe the habits of animals, both domesticated and wild, and in those days, mankind was living closer to nature and using none of today's processed foods. I am 84 years young, and see that it's quite difficult for this present generation to realize how the pioneers existed and thrived with few fatal degenerative illnesses such as cancer.

In any "health" profession, the practitioner has a good opportunity to observe the results obtained by the various modalities of treating the physical defects of patients. It's estimated that 85% of our learning is acquired through our eyes.

When I got out of college and started to practice my profession of fitting glasses, I soon realized that there must be an underlying cause for so much myopia (nearsightedness), cataracts, glaucoma, etc. As I gave the subject more study, it was clear to me that man was creating most of his eye problems by incorrect diet and poor choice of foods. For this reason, I took several courses in naturopathy and studied and read everything I could find in health books and magazines that dealt with the subject.

Many of my patients are so nearsighted that they are unable to see 20/20 on the eye chart. It's quite common for them to blame watching television and thus avoid the real cause, which is faulty diet and junk foods. Through the science of iridology, it's quite easy to observe unhealthy body conditions as well as deposits of drugs. I always try to emphasize basic health principles such as the importance of proper diet and tell my patients to avoid sugar, soft drinks and refined foods. Some will listen and, if they do, in a very short time their eyesight will improve. I've even had cases where I was then able to reduce the strength of the lenses.

One patient, age 75, had cataracts. I sent her to an ophthalmologist, who told her she'd have to have surgery in 3 months. I told her of Dr. Kelley's Nutritional Program and my wife, who's one of Dr. Kelley's technicians, had her evaluated. She followed the program and when she returned to the ophthalmologist, he told her she'd never have to have the surgery.

Another patient quite suddenly lost 70% of her eyesight. She went on Dr. Kelley's Nutritional Program and in a matter of 6 weeks, her eyesight returned.

When Dr. Kelley says we have been starving for 30 years, I certainly agree for I'm in a position to observe this. Dr. Kelley's no less than 75 years ahead of his time. Although this book deals primarily with cancer, that's by no means the limit to his concepts and abilities. I've seen many of the patients with other degenerative disease respond equally as well as the cancer patients."

Lloyd H. Price, O.D.
Des Moines, IA

Dr. Jack O. Taylor (Doctor of Chiropractic)

"I'd always held nutrition of some importance and often gave my patients rather inconsistent advice about 'improving your diet' or "why not try this vitamin for that symptom?' After several years of dealing with sick people, some of whom I knew were on good diets and some junk eaters, I began to realize that we were healthy not solely as a result of our intake, but instead, we were healthy or sick as a result of what our bodies did with the intake. It was discouraging to suggest the same "balanced" diet for several patients, getting entirely nowhere with many and having dramatic positive responses from others. Searching through the available literature seemed to add to my questions rather than provide answers.

Several years ago a dear friend developed cancer and my wife was invited to accompany her to see Dr. William Donald Kelley. Like many others, I'd heard of the success of Dr. Kelley in working with cancer patients and at that time could think of his nutritional program only as a cancer therapy. After meeting Dr. Kelley and observing his simple, systematic investigation of the individual body chemistry of our friend, my wife telephoned from Grapevine, Texas and insisted that I immediately come meet this man, as she knew his logical approach and reasonable conclusions would appeal to me. Early the next morning I was 1,100 miles from the luxurious surroundings of my suburban Chicago office, seated in a tiny frame house in a small Texas town. I forgot my surroundings, however, as I soon realized that here was a man who not only was answering my questions but was re-opening doors in my mind that had long been shut.

As I because better acquainted with Dr. Kelley, I soon realized that any help his Metabolic Medicine's Cancer Cure program gave to cancer patients was incidental to the balancing of their individual body chemistry. I began to apply these principles as 'nonspecific metabolic assistance' to meet my patient's individual needs. These programs have been so successful in helping gain and maintain health for many that I'd like to call your attention to the "non-cancer" aspects of Metabolic Medicine's concepts such as Dr. Kelley's Self-Test for the Different Metabolic Types. I consider it my privilege to encourage you to carefully study this book and expand your horizons of good health."

Jack O. Taylor, D.C.
Arlington Heights, IL

Dr. Richard Rovin (Naturopathic Doctor)

"This book is for those who have a strong belief in the principles that the body can heal itself and that nutrition is one of the keys to that healing. Nutrition has never before been approached as systematically and as aggressively as by Dr. Kelley. I was originally attracted to the field of Naturopathy because of my belief in our natural healing forces, and it's the same belief that has given me faith in this type of approach.

Food is more than separate nutritional factors; rather, it's a combination of nutrients that keep our body chemistry balanced and our organs in harmony and functioning optimally. So taken one step further, it's used not only to prevent disease or degeneration but, important to many of us, it may be used for regeneration and the removal of disease.

This new book will show that Dr. Kelley is constantly perfecting his work so it may help the most difficult cases and shed light on our biochemical individuality. This is truly the most important key to the development of a successful health program and why this book offers an avant-garde concept for today's health needs.

Doctors from all the professions are searching for the "magic bullet" that will prevent disease and maintain health. Some expect to find it in a synthetic drug and others in a particular natural substance, but the search is in vain, for we must appreciate our body's holistic needs and one agent alone cannot satisfy this. This approach considers nutrients for all the body's systems.

I anticipate further insights into people's well-being and greater health benefits for those who that follow and use the information in this book. Superior health services are already available to us. The IHI founded by Dr. Kelley is the first fruit of this research. Later, I expect these methods of analysis to act as a bridge between the different professions for the betterment of mankind.

It's a great joy to be part of this advanced system of healing. I appreciate the honor Mr. Rohé has afforded me by asking me to share my thoughts. I believe I represent my profession when I say that we're grateful to the past achievements of Dr. Kelley and cheer on and support future successes."

Richard Rovin, N.D.
Waialua, HI

Appendix II

Facts about Olestra

What do the experts say about olestra? Following are quotes from prominent doctors and scientists.

- "Olestra = Mineral oil. I believe this is another hoax and deception being foisted on the American people." Dr. Sheldon Margen, <u>Public Health Nutrition</u>, U. of California. Berkeley.
- "Olestra would constitute a public health time-bomb." Dr. John S. Bertram, Cancer Research Center of Hawaii (U. of Hawaii).
- "This substance has the potential to do significant harm." Dr. Ernst J. Schaefer, U.S. Department of Agriculture Human Nutrition Research Center on Aging, Tufts University.
- "We are concerned about the high incidence of gastrointestinal effects, ranging from diarrhea to fecal urgency, that are caused by the consumption of modest levels of olestra." Dr. Mark Donowitz, Johns Hopkins University School of Medicine.
- "It would be inappropriate to approve the use of olestra at this time." Dr. Mark Hegsted, Harvard Medical School and former Chief of Human Nutrition at the Department of Agriculture.
- "The bowel disturbances and impaired absorption of fat-soluble vitamins, including carotenoids, are sufficient reasons to have serious reservations about this food additive and to recommend that it not be introduced as a food additive." Dr. Ian Greaves, University of Minnesota School of Public Health.
- "It is clear folly to introduce this product into the diet of children." Dr. Herbert Needleman, University of Pittsburgh School of Medicine.
- "There are too many unanswered questions remaining about the safety and long-term public health consequences of olestra consumption. Therefore, the American Public Health Association does not support approval of olestra at this time." Dr. Fernando Trevino, American Public Health Association.
- "Even low levels of harm should not be tolerated when introducing a new product into the food supply. For olestra, the harm appears substantial. We would argue strongly that the FDA should neither approve Olestra for use in foods, nor should it be allowed into the U.S. food supply." Drs. John D. Potter and Johanna Lampe, Fred Hutchinson Cancer Research Center, Seattle.
- "The adverse effects of (olestra) outweigh its potential benefits." Jerianne Heimendinger, Cancer Research Center, Denver and former director of the National Cancer Institute's 5 A Day for Better Health Program.
- "Olestra — even in limited use — can be potentially harmful to the public. I do not believe that our society can afford such a risk (of macular degeneration)." Dr. Norman Krinsky, Tufts University School of Medicine.
- "There is strong reason to suspect that the effects (of olestra) will include increases in cancer,

heart disease, stroke and blindness." Drs. Walter Willett and Meir Stampfer, Harvard School of Public Health (endorsed by 25 other nutrition experts).

- "These estimates clearly demonstrate that the magnitude of carotenoid reduction demonstrated in controlled feeding studies of olestra could potentially produce a large number of deaths annually and major morbidity in the U.S. population. We strongly encourage you (Dr. Kessler) to avoid submitting the U.S. population, including children and pregnant women, to a massive uncontrolled experiment with potentially disastrous consequences." Drs. Walter Willett and Meir Stampfer, Harvard School of Public Health.

Post Script

Surviving A Healthy Childhood

By Kimberly S. Kelley

Men occasionally stumble over the truth, but most pick themselves up and hurry off as if nothing happened.
        —Winston Churchill

"William D. Kelley, D.D.S." That's what I put in the space marked "Father" on the hundreds of forms I have had to fill out in my time. In the space marked "Father's Occupation," I put "Health Researcher." That's about all the information I volunteer, with, a darn good reason, though. To my frequent embarrassment, my father has managed to attain a certain degree of fame. Euphemistically, he can be said to be controversial. Those less kindly disposed toward him might use the term "infamous." In any case, I have always found it easier simply to avoid him as a topic of casual conversation.

When we lived in tiny Grapevine, Texas, everyone in town knew of my dad - - The dentist in the little yellow office on Worth Street who didn't appear to be practicing dentistry. His patients didn't come from across town; they flew in from across the country. And the people coming to see him were all so desperately ill; many of them were cancer patients, obviously on their "last legs." Just what was going on in the small office?

The Fort Worth Star Telegram answered that question in a "shocking expose," which set the town buzzing. Dr. Kelley, an orthodontist, was seeing cancer patients! Further, the "therapy" he suggested was largely a matter of altering the diets of his patients and giving them vitamins and such! The notion that an individual's diet might be a factor in a disease as serious as cancer was considered absurd, but only slightly less so than the idea of a dentist working with cancer patients in any capacity. The scandal instigated by this article was the first I remember. Unfortunately, it was not the last.

My father became involved in cancer research first as a patient. In the early 1960's life in this family was relatively normal. At that time we lived in Midland, the tumbleweed capital of Texas. Dad was practicing orthodontics, and his practice was thriving. He belonged to the local country club, the school board, and the Church of Christ. In his spare time he indulged his passion for "tinkering" by restoring antique cars. His pride and joy was named Twinkles, a 1923 Cadillac that ran like a top in response to his diligent and loving care.

I would like to think that my father, given a choice, wouldn't have changed much in his life. However, he wasn't given the option.

Dad became ill in 1963, and critically so by 1967. The physicians he saw in Midland and Odessa couldn't find anything physiologically wrong with him for quite some time. The fact that he was ill was undeniably apparent; he was so weak, he found it necessary to lie down at the office between seeing patients. After he suffered what appeared to be two heart attacks, a diagnosis was finally made. The situation, I have been told, was as follows: He had cancer of the pancreas and liver. As is usually the case the malignancy was in its final stages at the time of diagnosis. The doctor refused to operate, saying Dad would die on the table. He should "get his affairs in order" quickly; he could expect to live only a few months. The doctor took my mother aside to tell her that, in his opinion, two months was a more realistic time frame.

One of the many reasons cancer is such an effective killer is its ability to destroy completely the individual's will to live. The patient suffers overwhelming pain, and his prognosis is rarely very optimistic. Any strength he might possess to combat the disease is soon exhausted, and death ceases to be viewed as something to be avoided. In death, the pain will be gone. The patient will no longer be forced to face the people he loves and the sorrow his suffering has brought them. Death becomes a friend, not an adversary. My mother and grandmother Kelley have told me stories of how terrible a thing it was to watch.

Unfortunately (or fortunately) my mother had some more unpleasant news for him. Mom has always had a real talent with a credit card. Due to the fact that we were living heavily in debt, she had quietly allowed Dad's life insurance to lapse. His death would leave his wife and three young daughters destitute.

I imagine Dad was very angry. He had come to terms with dying, but this news surely obliterated any peace of mind he might have attained. At some point he made the decision to do whatever he could to live. I do not know from what source he found the strength to attempt the impossible. Maybe his anger provided the motivation. (After all, if he died, he would not be able to kill my mom!)

Instead of tinkering with Twinkles, Dad now began tinkering with himself. The doctors had offered him no hope and no help; his only option was to take his case into his own hands. He was not overly armed for the fight; one of his degrees is in biochemistry, and he knew of several people conducting innovative research in natural healing. His illness was so severe that, by trial and error, he was able to determine quickly what substances (food, vitamins, and/or minerals) swung the pendulum of his well-being in what direction. Virtually everything the rest of the family ate would make him wretchedly ill. I remember sitting down to fried chicken with mashed potatoes and gravy, while dad dined on vile-smelling liver. My sisters and I did not understand why he was eating this way; no one told us he was dying.

Anyway, Dad must have done something right. Two months came and went, and the next four followed suit. During this time (and for sometime after, to be sure), Dad was critically ill; and for the purposes of this paper and its space limitation, I have greatly simplified the things he did to get well. But the bottom line is still the same; he didn't die.

Word got around — boy did it get around! The parents of Dad's orthodontic patients started asking him for advice about their ills and those of their loved ones. And Dad naively dispensed it. I don't believe it ever occurred to him to do otherwise. Many of those asking his advice were friends or, at least, people he knew. He simply told them what he had done to help himself. He had "been there" and knew first-hand the agony a cancer patient experiences. Here were people in desperate need of help. If he knew something that might ease their pain at all, he felt it was his moral duty to tell them. And many of those who did what he said got well.

People came to see Dr. Kelley in increasing numbers, and they were not looking to have braces put on their kids' teeth. Since he had to earn a living for his family but still felt a moral obligation to help anyone he could, he wrote a slim booklet in 1969 entitled *One Answer To Cancer.* In it was the story of his personal encounter with malignancy and the theoretical explanation of the procedures he used in getting well.

After the publication of ***One Answer To Cancer***, things really started to happen. As you might imagine, the American Medical Association, the State Board of Dental Examiners, and a host of other health-oriented organizations began to get hostile. He endured a great deal of persecution during this time, and found himself in quite a dilemma. On one hand, the number of individuals seeking his help was increasing; on the other, charges of "practicing medicine without a license" were being leveled at him. Eventually, he began seeing cancer patients for a living and started charging for his services. However, he saw only those people whose doctors had referred their patients to him. He consulted with the individual as well as the physician involved, always working well within the law. At the last count with which I am familiar, he has worked with over 33,000 patients in this way.

Dr. Kelley's case load has always been predictably lopsided; until recently, the only patients who came to him did so after being advised that there was nothing left to do but buy their burial plots and make out their wills. They had tried everything else before coming to see him. It is really amazing that he was able to save any of them at all. A great many of those early patients are alive and well today, singing his praises to anyone who will listen. In the cases of those who he was not able to save, their quality of life was still drastically improved. Many who succumbed to their illnesses did so without the reality-distorting drugs they once took for pain relief. Noting this, many of their relatives became vocal supporters of my father's work as well.

Dad has helped blaze a trail; he has been a genuine pioneer in his field. I think the phrase "health food nut" must have been coined specifically to describe him. It is difficult now to remember how "far out" his concepts were considered in 1969. Just as women today take for granted the rights their forerunners worked so hard to win, it is easy to forget that Dad preached health foods and ecology long before it became "chic" to do so. When I was growing up, many of my friends asked me why I never had acne at all; I was too embarrassed to tell them. I must admit I am shocked to see things I was forced to consume and hid frantically (such as granola or carrot juice) become not only socially acceptable but socially desirable!

When friends came over to play with my sisters and me, there were no snacks we felt comfortable offering them. There was food in the house, to be sure, but nothing they might recognize. The milk in the refrigerator was raw goat's milk (from a goat in the backyard — that by itself caused a great deal of comment). My mother milled wheat to make her own flour to bake her own bread. Instead of sugar the sweetener our family used was blackstrap molasses. Carob brownies are terrific, but if I offered them, I would have to explain that chocolate was not allowed in our house. People thought my parents were crazy, and I didn't really disagree.

Moreover, it was not just that we *ate* differently, Dad used the members of our family as guinea pigs to check out every new theory he came across in his research. For instance, he had all the silver fillings taken out of my mouth and replaced with gold. There had been quite a bit of silver in there, so the procedure took a long time and was expensive; I did not understand why he wanted to do this, nor did I bother to ask for an explanation. Nothing Dad did at that time made sense to my sisters or me; we just rolled our eyes and did as we were told. Just within the last year, however, I have heard the news that the composition of silver fillings changes over time, sometimes producing the same symptoms as does mercury poisoning. This is just one example out of hundreds. I am still discovering on a daily basis just how much ahead of his time my father has been, and now I can appreciate the courage it must have taken to adhere to the truths he found.

Dr. Kelley has never refused any patient. His philosophy is: "Where there's life, there's hope."

When actor Steve McQueen came to him for help, he did not turn him away, although he knew that accepting the man as a patient was actually dangerous. McQueen had a rare form of cancer, mesothelioma, which, to date, is always fatal. Again, he had been told to "get his affairs in order" by every physician he had seen; they offered him no hope. All the medical community could offer Mr. McQueen was a short delay of the inevitable by using surgery and chemotherapy. Steve McQueen was not unlike the rebel and the fighter he portrayed on-screen. Rejecting the concept of lying in a hospital bed, passively awaiting death, he preferred to fight to live, even in the face of odds no one could deny. Too, he had seen his friends (specifically, John Wayne) undergo the procedures the doctors recommended. He wanted no part of the slow, painful mutilation that held no hope of survival.

The last thing anyone involved wanted was that the story of McQueen's illness and subsequent treatment be leaked to the press. McQueen himself did not want the public to know he was ill; the people surrounding him did not want the star to be linked with the controversial treatment he was receiving. Dad did not want to go public with a famous patient whose chances of survival were so slim. He knew that if he lost a patient of McQueen's stature, that particular death would be all the public would remember; the lives he had saved would be overlooked entirely.

But that bastion of American Journalism, ***The National Enquirer***, unearthed the story. Possessing an intense hatred for the tabloid, McQueen insisted that he be allowed to break the news before the ***Enquirer*** could go to press. He wanted to tell his fans about his illness himself.

Steve McQueen died November 7, 1980, from complications arising after surgery performed for the purpose of removing dead tumor masses.

The majority of the media never did get the story straight. They had a field day with Dr. Kelley. I will never forget watching the ***Today Show*** and seeing my father sit there, verbally brutalized by Tom Brokaw and Jane Pauley, watching him say virtually nothing in his own defense. He had known the probable outcome of the situation and took the abuse as if it were his due. In reality, all he had done was try, to the best of his ability, to help another human being who had no other avenue open. Tom Snyder gave him a fair hearing, and so did several others; but such was the exception, not the rule.

Dad received a great deal of unexpected support from his old patients and their relatives, and I will never forget that either. He was swamped with their calls, letters, and gifts. They stood up to be counted; but, unfortunately, no one really cared about the lives Dr. Kelley saved — Steve McQueen was dead.

ing research in natural healing. When people calling there discovered that my last name is "Kelley," I am in for an earful of praise for my father. They launch into hour-long dissertations about how wonderful Dr. Kelley is and how his work improved or saved lives of loved ones. It seems to be important to these callers that Dr. Kelley's daughter should understand and appreciate the magnitude of his work; they all take upon themselves the personal responsibility of informing me who he is and what he has done. He receives thousands of cards and presents each year from people he no longer remembers. They remember him, though, and are grateful for his help.

But no one is more grateful than I. My "healthy childhood" may have caused me a little embarrassment from time to time, but it has stood me in good stead. Dad has taught me to search for the truth, even if it means questioning what others readily accept. I will always be thankful that my father had the insight to find the truth and the courage to say so."

Dallas, Texas

Acknowledgments

To Fred Rohé, M.T.; creative aothor of the 1980 *Metabolic Ecology* and the 1982 *Dr. Kelley's Answer to Cancer*, the 1999 and 2001 editions of this work.

To Greg Stirling, publisher of the 1997 and 1999 editions of *One Answer to Cancer*. his deep concern for the health of our civilization is evidenced by his willingness to publish contrary to the wishes of the Establishment.

To Bonnie O'Sullivan, editor of the 1999 edition of *One Answer to Cancer*, carried forward to this edition, who carefully considered those of you who are plagued with serious questions and demand answers. You will be eternally indebted. Bonnie has searched through all the collections of documents about the Kelley Metabolic Medicine's Paradigm that she could find from Kansas, Texas, Washington, Pennsylvania, California, and Georgia and everywhere in-between to give you the answers you need and desire.

To Roy Abell; Albert Abrams; Jack Abrams; W.A. Albrecht, Ph.D.; Robert Atkins, M.D.; Robert F. Armeit, M.T.; Megdalia Arnan, M.D.; Dorothy Arnett; Robert E. Arnett; Douglas M. Baird, D.O.; Broda Barnes, M.D.; Ervin Barr, D.O.; Jack Barron; John Bastyr, N.D.; Howard H. Beard, Ph.D.; Rollin E. Becker, D.O.; Henry Bieler, M.D.; Loren Biser; Samuel Biser; Randly L. Black, M.T.; Anne Blair, D.C.; Jeffrey S. Bland, Ph.D.; Paul C. Bragg, N.D., Ph.D.; David L. Braman, D.C.; Wilma J. Bryan, D.C.; Paul A. Buck, Ph.D.; Johanna Budwig, Frank Buell; Dean Burk, Ph.D.; Denis Burkitt, M.D.; Elizabeth Carlile, M.T.; J.E. Carlile, D.C.; Peg Carpenter, Rachel Carsoin, Emmanuel Cheraskin, M.D.; Peter Barry Chowka, Ann Cinquina, Durwood N. Clader, M.D.; Linda Clark, Irl C. Clary, D.M.D.; Warren Clough, M.A.; Donald Cole, M.D.; Sharon Collard, M.T.; Pat Connolly, Ernesto Contreras, M.D.; Alan Cott, M.D.; John Courtney, Norman Cousins, William D. Currier, M.D.; Johan P. Dahler, D.D.S.; Adelle Davis; Major DeJarnette, D.C.; Kirkpatrick Dilling, J.D.; Bill Dixon, D.C.; Kurt W. Donsbach, Ph.D., D.Sc., N.D., D.C.; Rita A. Dorris, M.T.; Beverly Dotson, M.D.; Dan Dotson, M.D.; Ruth Drown, D.C.; Darrell DuFresne; Jack V. Echtler, M.T.; Teena D. Echtler, M.T.; Catharyn Elwood, Ray Evers, M.D.; Ben Feingold, M.D.; Wayne Fisher, William H. Fisher, D.D.S.; Betty J. Fowler, M.T.; Carlton Fredericks, Ph.D.; Sanford C. Frumker, D.D.S.; Ellen M. Garris, M.T.; Charlotte Gerson, Max Gerson, M.D.; Bob Gibson, M.D.; Gina Glaze, M.T.; M.L. Goetting, Ph.D.; Doris Goetzinger, Harold Goetzinger, Ralph T. Golan, M.D.; Joseph Gold, M.D.; George Goodheart, D.C.; Ed Goodloe, Garry F. Gordon, M.D.; Gio B. Gori, Ph.D.; Edward Griffin, Dennis Gronick, J.D.; Bruce Halstead, M.D.; Darrel Boyd Harmon, Ph.D.; Harold W. Harper, M.D.; Karen Harper R.N.; Fred Hart, Orville L. Hastings, M.D.; William H. Hay, M.D.; Galen Hieronymus, Raymond W. Hillyard, M.D.; Abram Hoffer, M.D.; Ida Honorof, Beatrice T. Hunter, Dorsey Ingram, Amy L. Jackson, Kristi A. Jackson, Laura Jackson, Willard C. Jackson, D.C. Jarvis, M.D.; Bernard Jensen, D.C.; Pat Judson, Carl Kelley, John Mark Kelley, Kimberly S. Kelley, M.T.; L.P. Kelley, B.A.; Velma B. Kelley, W.B. Kelley, W.R. Kelley, D.D.S.; Fred Klener, M.D.; Wm. Koch, M.D.; Ernst Krebs, Jr., D.Sc.; Elizabeth Kubler-Ross, M.D.; Ronald S. Kurtz, Ph.D.; C.W. Lane, Peggy Lane, Gena Larson, Joan L. Laufer, M.T.; Bill Lawrence, Sophie Lawrence, Ira D. Leavitt, J.D.; Franklyn E. Lee, C.P.A.; Royal Lee, D.D.S.; Marge Leinhauser, M.T.; Dennis R. Lia Braaten, D.C.; Virginia Livingston, M.D.; Evarts Loomis, M.D.; Beatrice McClam, M.T.; Karyn McCoy, M.T.; Pat McGrady, Jr.; John Mann, J.D.; J.J. Matonis, J.D.; W.B. May, D.D.S.; Robert Mendelsohn, M.D.; Raggon L. Meyer, D.D.S.; Gael R. Minton, M.S.W.; Tyree G. Minton, Ed.D.; Betty Lee Morales, N.C.; Carol A. Morrison, M.D., F.A.C.C.; Edna P. Myrick, Raymond E.

Myrick, Beverly Nadler, M.T.; Manuel D. Navarro, M.D.; John E. Nelson, D.C.; Russel Nelson, D.C.; Joe D. Nichols, M.D.; Hans Nieper, M.D.; Allan H. Nittler, M.D.; William F. Nolan, Gary Null, Kay Ortman, John Ott, D.Sc.; D.D. Palmer, Arthur s. Parker, D.M.D.; Richard Passwater, Ph.D.; F.M. Pottenger, Jr., M.D.; Inez Price, M.T.; Lloyd H. Price, O.D.; Weston A. Price, D.D.S.; James Privitera, M.D.; Grady Ragsdale, Wilhelm Reich, M.D.; Rodney Reinbold, J.D.; John. W. Rhinehart, M.D.; John Richardson, M.D.; Thomas Roberts, M.D.; Lorraine Rosenthall, Richard G. Rovin, N.D.; Luanne Ruona, M.D.; Ruth Sackman, Michael Schachter, M.D.; Emil K. Schandl, Ph.D.; W. Scheef, M.D.; D. Schildwaechter, M.D.; Milo Seiwert, M.D.; C. Norman Shealy, M.D.; David Shenkin, M.D.; Edward N. Siguel, M.D., Ph.D.; Carl Simonton, M.D.; Ada Mae Simpson, J.P. Simpson, Adele I. Smith, R.N.; Lendon Smith, M.D.; Robert H. Snow, M.D.; James F. Sommers; Jerry Spencer, D.C.; Joe Spruell, D.O.; Henry A. Stahr, D.C.; Horace Standlee; Sue Standlee; John R. Stanfield, D.O.; Sarah Starr, Cameron Stauth, Rachael Stevens, R.N.; Scott Stirling, Andrew T. Still, M.D.; William G. Sutherland, D.O.; Albert Szent-Gyorgyi, M.D.; John L. Tate, D.D.S.; Jack O. Tayler, D.C.; Esther Thaler, R.N.; E.E. Thompson, D.O.; Emory Thurston, Ph.D.; Jamie O'Shea Chastain, John W. Travis, M.D.; Lois Tubman, M.T.; Henry Turkel, M.D.; Carole Valentine, Tom Valentine, Robert B. Vance, D.O.; Norman W. Walker, D.Sc.; Charles Walters, Jr.; David S. Walther, D.C.; Otto Warburg, Ph.D.; Paul A. Wedel, M.D.; Richard Welch, M.D.; Juline L. Wenig, D.C.; Murrell Weston; Paul A. White, D.C.; Ann Wigmore, Ph.D.; Henry N. Williams, M.D.; Roger Williams, Ph.D.; Suzi Kelley Wolcott, M.T.; Mickey Wrathall, John Yiamoulannis, Ph.D.; Mary Maude Zilliox, M.T.; Royal Q. Zilliox, M.T.; and many others who with personal risk and expense have, down through the years, brought Metabolic Medicine's concepts to you through their creative writing and outstanding work.

Index

A

abnormal placenta **8**
acid/alkaline balance **11**, **24**, **39**, **51**, **60**
AIDS **24**, **131**, **132**
alcohol drink **32**
alfalfa **46**, **47**
Allergic Reactions **76**
allergies **20**, **140**, **141**
Almonds **48**
Alzheimers **113**
American Cancer Society **122**, **134**
amino acids **11**, **23**, **44**
Amylase **10**
Anglo-Saxon **11**
Anthrax **130**
anti-enzyme factors **11**
antibiotic-free **45**
antibiotics **104**, **137**
apple juice or cider **31**
Aryans **11**
Asians **12**
autonomic nervous system **11**, **59**, **60**

B

B. Anthraces **130**
backaches **33**
Bananas **48**
Beans **47**
beet **33**, **47**, **63**
Beta-Z **45**
bile flow **31**
biliousness **33**
Biological Warfare infections **132**
Biological Warfare Weapons **130**
Biologicals **11**, **130**, **132**
Biopsy **15**, **77**, **113**
biopsy **15**, **20**, **21**, **77**, **79**, **81**, **83**, **94**, **99**, **100**, **104**, **126**, **130**
Blacks **12**, **131**
Bladder **31**, **33**, **64**
blood supply **10**, **11**
bloodstream **8**, **31**, **39**, **88**
Body Detoxification **29**
Bone **65**, **102**, **135**
Bone Cancer **102**
bowel movement **36**, **37**, **66**
brainwashing **133**